Taken In Hand

A Guide to Domestic Discipline, Power Exchange Relationships,
and Related BDSM Topics

By Jolynn Raymond
Head of Household, Mistress, Dominant,
Wife, BDSM Advisor and Author

A Guide to Domestic Discipline,
Power Exchange Relationships,
and Related BDSM Topics
By Jolynn Raymond

Copyright November 2013
All Rights Reserved
Kindle Edition: Amazon
Paperback by Createspace
Edited by Rachel Scott
Cover design by Jolynn Raymond

Other Books by Jolynn Raymond

Lessons of Love: A Kinky Historical Romance
Elizabeth's Destiny: A Kinky Historical Romance
Sweet Agony: A Collection of Erotic BDSM Short Stories
Dining In: A Taste of Erotic Food Play
Dark Obsessions: A Collection of Lesbian BDSM Erotica

Paranormal Historical Romance Trilogy
Taken... Book One in the Beneath the Shadows of Evil
Torn... Book Two in the Beneath the Shadows of Evil
Treasured... Book Three in the Beneath the Shadows of Evil

Books Featuring the Connelly Witches
Shattered Images
A Past Undone

All books are available for electronic download/Kindle or
in paperback on Amazon.com

Websites
My Books on Amazon: *http://www.amazon.com/Jolynn-Raymond*
Jolynn Raymond's Dark Obsessions: *http://jolynnraymond.com*
Dark Obsessions is an informational/educational BDSM Forum
My fan page on Facebook: *https://www.facebook.com/JolynnRaymond*
Follow me on Twitter: *https://twitter.com/JolynnRaymond*

Disclaimer

I am not endorsing the punishment of anyone, especially children. I am stating how I like things to be run in my household, but that is me. What others do in their own homes is up to them. This book is intended for consenting adults only. I hold no responsibility for anyone's actions after reading this book. Proceed at your own risk. I am not liable. I do not recommend spanking without knowing a good deal about it, and knowing how an implement feels before you use it on someone. Communication beforehand is vital. Any actions done after reading this book are the sole responsibility of the reader. Be safe, sane, and consensual. Spanking someone without their consent is abuse.

Foreword

This book is intended to be a guide to help couples develop a domestic discipline or power exchange relationship, and as an introduction into the world of BDSM as it relates to some power exchange interactions. It is meant to provide insight to those who wish for their relationship to be a domestic discipline (DD) type without any BDSM aspects, as well as offering up the intricacies of domination and submission in conjunction with a power exchange relationship for those that choose that lifestyle. Regardless of the role you choose to take or the elements of kink you may wish to add to your relationship, learning about the things that interest you should always be the first step.

It is my hope that those who are interested in a solely domestic discipline run household will not shy away from this book because it contains information on BDSM. Each and every relationship is different no matter your religious beliefs, your views regarding kink, the gender of those involved, or the ways in which you see your relationship taking on a power exchange aspect. What gives integrity to a BDSM power exchange relationship gives that same integrity to a domestic discipline one. All require the person in charge to be safe, sane, non-abusive, and honorable. All of them also require the couple to be in agreement, and must include consent for what is to become the structure of their life together.

The dominant or head of household, must inform the person who will be on the receiving end of the discipline before any type of commitment, marriage, or collaring, and well ahead of the first punishment. To not inform someone is extremely misleading and as such turns any discipline into abuse. If you are in a long standing relationship and are now looking to add domestic discipline, you must have a conversation with your significant other before a domestic discipline plan is put in place. The ideal plan has input from both of the people involved. Being the head of household or dominant should not be akin to being a dictator.

As stated above, and this does need repeating, if you don't have consent, it is abuse. I feel this goes for Christian domestic discipline as well. Your religion may say it is your right as a husband to punish your wife if she doesn't obey, but simply telling her she will be disciplined as you see fit, and then instituting a relationship that is based on obedience and punishment is a misuse of authority. The one who will be subjected to punishment must have a chance to refuse or object; otherwise it does not fall under the act of giving consent, especially if you have been married for a long while. If you decide your relationship would be made stronger by adding domestic discipline, it must be agreed upon. There is a very distinct line between domestic discipline and abuse. Please do not cross it, whichever type of relationship you have.

Table of Contents:

Introduction
Why Did I Choose Domestic Discipline?
My Domestic Discipline Marriage
Life in My Domestic Discipline Household
Building an Ethical Domestic Discipline Relationship
Creating an Outline for the TiH
The Inevitable First Punishment
The Importance of Bonding, Communication, and Nurturing
Pitfalls, Disillusionment, Burnout, and Mistakes
How to Punish Ethically and Effectively
Keeping a Domestic Discipline Relationship Free of Abuse

Topics That Pertain to BDSM as well as DD, and Power Exchange

The Different BDSM, DD and Power Exchange Roles
So You Think You Want to Be a Dominant
You Think You're Submissive. Now What?
The Power Exchange of Service Submission
Pre Service Checklist and Rules Prior to Becoming My Submissive
How to Approach a Mistress
How to Approach a Submissive and the Idea of the Submissive Slut
Anal Sex Tutorial/ How to introduce Anal Sex
Understanding the Appeal of Spanking
Styles and Reasons for Spanking
The Ins and Outs of BDSM Gatherings
Power Exchange Means Give and Take

Introduction

When people pick up an advice book they often wonder what makes the author knowledgeable enough to write about a subject. While I don't have a psychology degree that grants insight into how people react and what makes them tick, I do have a job that requires me to be well schooled in behavior modification and human nature. I have been the head of my household in loving DD relationships for close to fifteen years. Simply put, I know what works. Much has been fined tuned after trial and error, and different relationships have made it clear that a cookie cutter approach can't be relied upon. Each couple who ventures into DD, or power exchange, is different, and therefore the structure of the relationship must be created specifically for each couple. The approaches in this book are guides to build the foundation of a healthy relationship, as well as providing suggestions for when things seem to go off track.

The subjects of this book are often geared towards the dominant or head of the household in the relationship, but the submissive or the one who is taken in hand in a power exchange relationship can learn about how best to establish a domestic discipline lifestyle as well. There are safety tips, cautions about the wrong kind of people projecting themselves as dominants, and guidelines I have set for my submissive wife contained within these pages. This book is not exclusively for the dominant. Perhaps if one is bold enough, they can leave a copy of this book on their partners desk or nightstand to let them know about the desire to make their relationship one in which the more dominant partner takes the lead.

The following abbreviations will be used in this book:

- DD – Domestic Discipline
- HoH – Head of Household
- TiH – Taken in Hand (the person who is subjected to discipline/or submits to it)
- BDSM – Bondage, Discipline, Sadism, and Masochism, or as some prefer the S and M can stand for submissive and Master.
- D/s – Dominant/submissive

The word dominant will be used for either a male or female just as submissive can be either gender. Some believe that a domestic discipline home can only be run by a male. I, of course, don't buy into that train of thought. Granted my wife and I are a same-sex couple, but I know of several female run households where the submissive or TiH is a male. Gender has little to do with dominance just as submission has little to do with being male or female.

My qualification to write a Domestic Discipline and BDSM tutorial comes from reading, experiencing trial and error in my own relationships, and being active in BDSM and the kink community for quite a few years. In that time I have learned techniques, been schooled in protocol, have immersed myself in the kink community and the wealth of information it provides, as well as establishing good relationships with those in the community who are ethical leaders. I observe, have conversations, attend seminars and conventions, ask questions, and go forward with the attitude that one should never stop learning.

I have found the love of my life and we have a happy and fulfilling domestic discipline relationship. I never want that to change. We will grow and evolve as a couple, but it is my hope that through communication, discipline, trust, and love, my wife will always be by my side. Relationships that don't grow become stagnant. Ones that take a proactive stance to have a set plan to maintain a solid structure, and a system of accountability, discipline, and forgiveness, can provide the stability it takes to weather the stressors of life.

My views are often lofty and serious, for I believe that one must always be well informed and put their partner first. This view is not always well received, and I have been in many debates concerning the treatment of those who are submissive. BDSM doesn't have to be serious stuff as long as there is respect and consent for everyone. At times I am known to get very ridiculous when I play. What those of us who are into BDSM do for recreation is supposed to be fun and enjoyable. I'm all for that, as long as the dominant or top in a scene has the best interest of the submissive or bottom at heart.

Why Did I Choose Domestic Discipline?

There has been a lot of negative press concerning domestic discipline as of late, so I want to address the whys of dominance, while at the same time answer questions that people who are just starting out often have. I'm also speaking about why I personally am dominant, because if you are thinking about becoming the head of a domestic discipline household or the dominant in a D/s power exchange relationship, you need to be able to clarify just what it is that you think makes you qualified to be in charge of not just your life, but the life of your partner. I'm not saying that to challenge anyone, I'm saying it because you need to be clear on the reasons why you wish to live this sort of lifestyle, and understand all it entails. There are things about DD relationships and BDSM roles that I wasn't aware of when I first started out, and they made a big difference in creating the dominant woman I am today.

When I wasn't into kink, or thought I wasn't, my personality could have been called bossy or in some instances, bitchy. I hate that line of thought, though. Just because I stand up for what I believe in and fight for my family and friends and what I feel is right, it doesn't make me a bitch, and being dominant doesn't make me a bitch either. There are many traits that come through in people who hold the power in a power exchange relationship, and there really is no wrong or right, aside from having the consent of the person you are involved with, treating people with respect, and taking your role as protector seriously.

There are something like six types of dominant people according to the books. They run from a dominant who does not necessarily thinks of themselves as god, but wants to be worshipped and be the all and everything to their slave, submissive, or domestic partner, to the nurturing parental dominant who wants to do all for their little (adult) girl or boy. In between there are dominants that encompass everything from being very strict, maintaining high protocol, being nurturing, harsh, quiet, loud and demanding, and pretty much everything you can wrap up into the personality of someone who has a need to be in charge and have things go their way.

When I put that into words it sounds selfish, but there is a difference between a spoiled diva, a guy who wants a sex slave to boss around, and a proper head of household. Dominant people who engage in consensual power exchange relationships have their partner's best interest at heart, or else they damn well should. I do, so the whole 'doing things my way' issue has been talked over and agreed upon. Beauty knew this before I married and collared her. She gave me consent.

There are a lot of things you may read or hear depending on what type of dominant is offering advice. A submissive must always take care of their dominant. A dominant must always control themselves; a dominant is all about a me, me, me personality; a good dominant is strict, a good dominant keeps their s type on their toes, again, there are a lot of things said about the 'true' way or as it's commonly called when we are rolling our eyes, the 'twue' way. What it boils down to is what works for each individual.

There are people who think a slave or submissive should sleep on the floor, never speak unless spoken to, and always sit at their feet. They are a bit too extreme for me. Others think I'm nuts for actually having discussions with my wife and allowing her to have an opinion, allowing her to be clothed when we are in our home, and cuddling and so forth, but again, their beliefs don't work for me. The chasm between us is huge, but that isn't to say how they do things or how I do things is wrong.

I did much soul searching when I had my eyes opened to the fact that, hell yes I am dominant, and dominant isn't a bad thing. Being a sadist took a lot longer, but that said, I DID come to terms with them both. Why and how? Because all of my relationships are consensual, there is no abuse even when I do a heavy impact play session. I care about my partners (non-sexual BDSM play). I cherish my wife. I care about her very much, and taking care of her, disciplining her, giving her structure and outlining her life, grounds the both of us.

I receive the absolute control I crave and need in this crazy world by living as the head of household in a domestic discipline relationship. It's my rock in a world where I can't have everything my way. In our home, in our relationship, I am in charge, period. I like things done the way I like them done. I like X,Y,Z to be ready or prepared when I come home. When it isn't done, there is a consequence. It's what Beauty wants in a relationship. She doesn't have to make decisions, I do that. She doesn't have to worry about the little things in life; I try to take care of them.

I am not a dominant who is always in complete control. I am human. Ours is a 24/7 lifestyle marriage and we are both menopausal, so yes, I get irate at times, but I never punish in anger. I am not perfect, she is not perfect. I don't expect her to be and she knows I'm not. Ours is a give and take relationship, but yes, I am in charge. I also want to let you know that being the dominant is hard work. I choose to take on the world and deal with the crap life flings at us in exchange for being taken care of in our home. For us it's a good power exchange.

My Domestic Discipline Marriage

I am currently the head of household in a domestic discipline marriage; the fact that we are kinky in no way means we are sexually promiscuous or non-monogamous to each other. I am in no way attempting to pass judgment on those who are poly, I am simply stating that all of my adult relationships that have included an element of power exchange and loving domestic discipline have been monogamous.

My marriage would be considered a 1950's style type of DD. My wife doesn't work outside of the home. She is my treasured housewife and the love of my life. In this book she will be referred to as Beauty, which is part of her name on Fetlife.com. It is her job to take care of the pets, the house, and tend to all the details that are an annoyance to me. She is expected to carry out any tasks given to her as well as follow the schedule that has been set. It is also her job to create a place of serenity for me to come home to each day after work.

I did not just jump into the role of head of household and dominant. Dominance, while somewhat innate, is not something you can simply do without the knowledge that will make you an ethical HoH, Mistress, or Master. One must be reasonable, grounded, safe and sane. Sitting and ordering a spouse, submissive, or slave about, or wielding the power to spank your wife or husband for not doing something you want is not all there is to it. You must have a genuine concern for the other person's well-being. They are giving themselves and their life up to you.

Controlling another person's life is a big responsibility. Be you a Christian couple who believe that the man in a marriage should make all the decisions and rule with an iron fist, a powerful woman who knows it is her place to be in control, a strict no-nonsense disciplinarian or a nurturing dominant, your partner comes first. They do as you wish and see to your needs, and therefore you must see to all of theirs.

No matter what you want to explore or what role you wish to take, knowing the difference between abuse, fantasy BDSM, and reality is vital. BDSM movies and books rarely portray real relationships, or show the important act of aftercare and the forgiveness that must be given when showing a punishment spanking scene. No one ever knows it all. I am a huge advocate for hands on learning and exploring relationships with knowledgeable people. While I always encourage people to get involved in their kink community, I know that isn't always possible. It is my hope that this guide can help those interested in DD and/or BDSM to navigate the waters, despite the different viewpoints of my readers. Start smart and stay aware.

It is important to note that the fact that I am sadistic in some of my BDSM play in no way relates to my DD marriage. My wife is somewhat of a masochist and we do engage in pleasurable or 'funishment' spankings and impact play, but the discipline that is involved in our domestic discipline marriage has nothing to do with my sadistic trait. I get absolutely no pleasure in punishing my wife.

This guide hardly covers everything, and I do not claim to know it all or intend to say that my ways and beliefs are the only way. This is simply the way I do things. How I train, how I instruct, and how I discipline has been learned over time, and is what fits best for me. I differ greatly from many in the lifestyle who view the line between Master and slave as something that can't be crossed, and also from many of the Leather Community Masters. I don't believe that only a man can be the dominant or that a dominant female must have masculine mannerisms. There is a 'true' way of doing things, but I do respect protocol and the right others have to run their DD or power exchange relationships different from mine. The only thing that must be a constant in any relationship is the fact that anyone considering being a dominant must be ethical in their intent and actions.

    Discover what works for you. No two people are alike. Your beliefs may not be another's beliefs, and your kink may not be another's kink, but that's okay. Ideals change, limits change, people change as we learn and grow. This guide is intended as learning tool, a place to start, and a tutorial on how to begin. You can learn from my mistakes and discoveries instead of starting from scratch. Caution must be used no matter what type of lifestyle you decide is right for you, and you and your partner must communicate. Always be safe, be knowledgeable, and have consent. A loving domestic discipline or power exchange relationship that is long lasting is possible. It just takes respect and communication from those at the heart of it.

Life in My Domestic Discipline Household

To get an idea of what my domestic discipline household looks like, you might want to imagine a home in the 1950's or for those of you who are older like me, a "Leave It to Beaver" style family minus the dress and pearls, and plus a hairbrush in the nightstand for spankings. Often the kink couples who like the 1950's household intermingle with the domestic discipline folks, but not always. Mine has shades of the 1950's because we are the old style, traditional home where one partner works outside the home, or is the breadwinner, and sets the rules and tone of the household, and one stays home to tend the house and kids. In this day and age, it isn't always financially possible to have one person stay at home. Even so, the home can be run in a domestic discipline manner.

As stated above, the main abbreviations you will often find in articles or discussions about domestic discipline homes are DD – which is simply domestic discipline, HoH – which is head of household (which in our case is me), and TiH – which means taken in hand. This is the person on the receiving end of the discipline and who typically doesn't make the rules. My wife Beauty is the TiH in our home, and though she is allowed to give her opinion on how things are run and make requests for things we need outside of her monthly budget, I make the final decisions. That said, I do not wish to have a robotic wife or a meek and docile woman who doesn't speak unless spoken to, has no opinions of her own, and strives only to be perfect for the HoH. We are both real people with emotions and intelligence.

I desire a partner to laugh with and be a good conversationalist. I want to hear her opinions, and I love that she has an odd sense of humor. If we were both vanilla, meaning not into kink, we would still be a good match. She is obedient most of the time, and does a great job taking care of me, our home, and our pets. She desires to be submissive to me. There is no force involved, and I wouldn't be happy if there were. I am not one who wants a relationship with a woman who must be made to do the things that are commanded. Some dominants or HoH's do, and enjoy the taming and constant power struggle needed to keep their partner in line, but that type of relationship isn't for me.

All of the things mentioned here are very important issues to take into consideration if you wish to develop a DD or power exchange relationship. Think about your needs and those of your partner or potential partner. Think about outside interests. If you wish to have a stay at home wife you need someone who can be content with that kind of life. If you wish for a woman or partner who has a high level of power in their job but comes home and is submissive, then again, you must find someone who can do that. You need to be a match, DD or BDSM wise, in your home, but also have things in common as just people.

I make the rules for how our home is to be run, but the rules are a fluid document. That doesn't mean they change all the time at my whim. That would make the expectations I put forth for Beauty to follow impossible to live up to. A strong DD relationship must have a solid foundation, and ours does. What I mean by fluid is that over time things come up and needs change on both sides of the spanking spoon. Your ideals may change over time as the needs of your submissive partner change and you grow as a couple. My high expectations as to how clean the house is to remain, what the food budget is for the month, what Beauty's allowance is, what extras may be bought, how I wish to be welcomed home, and really all of our routines from simple and ordinary to complex are mostly unchanging. That said, they are decided by me with thought given to Beauty's current capabilities. Outside stressors such as family, health issues, and other random needs cause changes that a good HoH or dominant is flexible enough to take into consideration.

    I have a particular way that I like things to be done. For example, the bed is to be turned on (we have a heated mattress pad), my water bottle filled, the bedside light turned on, all about an hour before I go to bed. In our case while we were in the training period of our relationship, my wife learned how I expected our home be kept, personal duties for me such as doing my nails, what foods I enjoy, how much she is to spend on groceries, and all the little things that make our house a home. Training my wife took time. Do not expect things to be perfect right away. We learn by mistakes. I will talk more about this later in the section on pitfalls.

    A schedule to help her with when things are expected to be done has been alternately given out on a daily and weekly basis so Beauty knows what is expected for the day. Some routines are bi weekly, weekly, and other routines are done daily. She greets me at the door with a kiss, has my tea ready, and is ready to listen if I need to vent about my day. She serves me dinner at a specific time, makes sure I have something to drink at all times when I am home, and knows she is expected to clean up right away after dinner. I know this sounds odd to some and like she waits on me hand and foot, but as the breadwinner and dominant, this is how we run things. We both want this.

As the TiH, Beauty must do as I have instructed. This type of lifestyle and the things I demand of her were agreed upon when we became a couple, and became a permanent part of our lives when I collared and married her. She said that she would abide by my rules and wishes. She has given her consent for punishment and is in full agreement to living in a DD household. The vows Beauty said included obey, and she does. She has obligations that must be adhered to or there are consequences. These consequences are clearly spelled out and were discussed prior to our marriage and prior to the first punishment she ever received. My wife is not abused, she is disciplined. The difference between the two is huge. Her consent means everything.

Some of the tasks she does to keep our home running smoothly and make it a place where I can come home to serenity are as follows:

- She keeps a list of groceries we need. Running out of things we need isn't an option. She also has a budget and is expected to stay within it. She has an allowance, but any spending outside of it or her budget must be cleared with me.

- Once she is told of upcoming events that may change our schedule or require extra duties for her, she is to adjust and make it work.

- She is to keep track of my book ads, upcoming events, book giveaways and promotions.

- She is expected to do most if not all of the errands that need doing, such as take the pets to the vet, go to the pharmacy, the post office, getting gas, and taking the car in for any needed maintenance.

- She has a schedule of when the bathrooms are to be cleaned, the linens changed, the floors done, the house vacuumed, when to dust, when to do laundry, etc. The following links can help the TiH get organized so the house is always clean, the meals on the table on time, the groceries bought, and so on.

Beauty has worked with Cozi and Fly Lady. She struggles and has difficulties managing her time. Both websites provide support for staying organized and keeping a clean house.

http://www.flylady.net

http://www.cozi.com

    As a submissive, she wants this type of control. It's comforting. As I said, she has trouble managing her time and the structure of our DD household is something she needs and desires. It makes it possible for her to be free of decision making. She has a time which she is to get up by, and most of the time she goes to bed when I do. She is expected to take care of herself by taking all her meds, eating right (for the most part), telling me of any physical problem that might require a visit to the doctor or dentist, telling me if she needs something, etc.

    Beauty is also to tell me if something has upset her or if she is struggling for any reason. It is then my job to figure out how to solve the problem. We live a lifestyle where she takes care of me and I take care of us. We do not have kids that are still at home, but many DD couples do. The children do know of our relationship style. They are old enough now (24 and 28), and the oldest is in the kink lifestyle. Neither was ever exposed to DD or kink as children, and I would never discipline Beauty while they were at the house. The workings of our DD relationship are carried out in private.

    DD couples with children still at home must, in my opinion, carry out any punishment in a way that the children are not aware of it. I do not approve of the children being subjected to seeing their mom or dad disciplined. It is my view that children could misconstrue what is seen. It could lead to fear of the HoH, and the loss of respect by the children for the TiH. When they are adults they can make their own decisions be it from the teaching of a church, an interest in the BDSM lifestyle, or simply following the structured ways of the home they were raised in. Exposure to seeing their mother kick and cry as she is being paddled or strapped has the potential for too many pitfalls. It demeans the mother or TiH and could start a vicious cycle of abuse. The adults involved understand the element of consent, children cannot.

Building My Ethical Domestic Discipline Relationship

      The first thing needed to build a strong foundation for domestic discipline in any relationship, whether it's new or seen as a positive change for an existing one, is open and honest communication. If you are currently without a partner you need to make a list of the things that you would consider vital to any relationship you enter into so you can keep the list at the forefront of your mind when meeting potential partners. I am all for going to munches organized by the local kink community if you are single but wish for a DD or power exchange relationship. This doesn't mean go to a munch solely to find a partner, it means go to meet others with the same mindset. The kink community is like any other in regards to friends knowing of friends who would be a great match up.

      You have a much better chance of finding someone who shares your views at an event for those who are into BDSM. Searching online is difficult at best because of all the pretenders, and the regular or vanilla nightlife in whatever city or town you are in, doesn't cater to a group of people are specifically open minded about kink. Munches are simply a gathering of kink friendly people in a vanilla setting. It's all very much like going out to dinner or drinks except those present are more apt to have the same desires as you do. Munches aren't hook up events and you should attend simply to make friends. Go to learn, go to meet people, and go with an attitude of respect. Be open minded in regards to other's kink, behave in the way you would when meeting a vanilla partner. Kinky does not equate to promiscuous, and don't expect submissive people to call you Sir or Ma'am.

Am I saying you shouldn't start a relationship with someone who doesn't agree with your relationship needs? Yes I am, and I'll stick by that conviction. If you strongly believe that you need to be the HoH or dominant person in your relationship or if you feel you need to be in a relationship with someone who is comfortable taking control and punishing you if needed, then you need to stick with your ideals. Trying to push someone into a domestic discipline relationship will be frustrating instead of fulfilling, and can, in the worst case scenario, lead to accusations of abuse. I've seen people try to be vanilla because they love their partner or have met someone they really like, but I have never seen someone feel complete without a partner who shares their beliefs.

If you are already in a relationship and wish to add a DD aspect, it can be very hard to open the door on that particular conversation, but communication is the only way to see eye to eye. The HoH or dominant, and the one taken in hand or who is submissive, have to agree on the aspects of the relationship. Chastising someone, punishing them, trying to control all they do is abusive unless you have their consent. Let me say that again. Punishing someone physically and trying to dictate every aspect of their life without their consent is abuse. I know I keep saying that, but it is vitally important. You should make up a list of expectations that are clear and consistent as well as what the consequences for failure to do things are. The HoH must list their responsibilities as well. Types of punishment must be accepted and agreed to, as well as respecting your partner's limits or their request that something in particular never be done.

Regardless of why you are interested in building a DD or power exchange relationship, there are some basic principles and ethical considerations that must be considered. When I entered into a relationship with my wife and subsequently married and collared her, I made her promises about how I would care for her and always take her needs into consideration. She in turn promised to obey me. That is a promise that doesn't come easily. Her promise meant she was giving up her free will in order to allow me to make decisions for her. Beauty was able to do that because she trusts me to always strive to do my best for her. Her submission and the power it gives me should never be abused. Her promise to obey doesn't mean I get carte blanche to create rules on a whim, punish just because I feel like it or am in a bad mood, disregard her needs in favor of mine, or in general abuse my authority.

Below is a list I gave my wife when we first entered into a dominant and submissive relationship. I was told once, when I posted it on Fetlife.com, that it would get me kicked out of the Dominant's Union. It was said in a joking manner, but in all seriousness, my view of how things should be done and the promises I make, are not always the norm. I understand that and your mileage may vary.

I believe respect is a two-way street and that my wife is as important as I am in our relationship. It's not just about me. She may be responsible for making sure my wishes are carried out, but I am responsible for her. Any good DD, CDD, or power exchange relationship must consider both parties, and everyone's needs must be addressed. Whether you feel my ethics and promises are over the top, or right on the mark, please act in a way that is protective and ethical as well as structured and strict.

In my mind the things listed below are things that need to be thought out and adhered to, or at the least have some form of them in place. They are a code of ethics I vow to abide by. They are what I view as vital for us to be a loving and committed Mistress/submissive, DD, and married couple. I feel they are an intricate part of a strong domestic discipline relationship because the one in charge MUST always govern themselves and take responsibility for the person they have power over.

- *I will always respect your safeword immediately and will never attempt to make you feel shame for saying it. NEVER. It is your only out and that one word will cease any and all actions at once so we can discuss what's going on.* – When Beauty is punished, I would accept her safeword, but when she is punished she knows the reason, and therefore I doubt she would ever use the word that would stop her punishment. Still, she has that option. If she were to safeword, I would punish her in a different way after we discussed why she said it. To date, this has never happened.

- *I will never punish or strike you in anger. If I am displeased or angry I will remove myself from the situation until my anger has passed and I can deal with whatever has caused my anger in a calm manner. Punishments (except corner time) will only be done in a loving and protective manner.*

- *I will always listen to your point of view or desires without judgment. I have the final say in all matters dealing with punishment, pain, and pleasure, but I will always listen and then explain my decision.*

- *I will always treat you with respect as the valued person you are. I may own you, treat you as my whore during a play scene, call you nasty filthy names, use you in all sorts of manner that bring us both pleasure, but it will be on a mutually wanted basis and I will never be demeaning to you as a person or attempt to crush your self-esteem.*

- *We will never do something in a play session that could harm you in a serious manner. This does not mean I will not push your limits. I will and plan to, but I will not break the skin, cause bleeding, force you to hold a position that is causing your hands or feet to become numb, etc. Pain yes, injury never. *One note. I know plenty of couples who do play hard and skin is broken, but there is aftercare and all precautions are taken to tend any cuts or wounds. I am not saying that causing bleeding is bad practice, it simply isn't my thing.*

- *I will always respect "No, I do not want to play (or have sex) today." That does not mean you can get out of a punishment, it simply means I understand you may not always be feeling sexual or want D/s, so we will wait.*

- *If I walk away to calm down, I will always come back. This relationship will not end without doing everything in our power, including counseling, to communicate and fix what isn't working.*

- *I will hold you to your rules and call you on your misbehavior in order to give you the much needed structure in your life.*

- *I will protect you, nurture you, love you, punish you, support you, and do all in my power to help you stay centered and deal with the things in your life that cause you pain.*

- *I will not break this code of ethics.*

Whether you agree with these specific promises or have different views, you must embrace some kind of ethics if you are going to take on the control of and responsibility for someone else's life. The ease and temptation to abuse your power must be tempered by some sort of vow that your wife/submissive/partner can hold you to with the intent of helping to keep you grounded and keep your power in check.

I readily admit that I don't always abide by my own lofty expectations and promises. I'm one who raises my voice too often, and I fuss instead of taking immediate action when I am tired, so it helps that these promises are written and can be read from time to time by both my wife and I. I'm human, and my wife knows that. In turn I must always remember that my wife is human too. We are not infallible. I've had far too many debates with dominants who believe that their submissive must be in service mode and be ready to submit to anything including sexual submission despite anything that's going on with them, and it makes me wonder how on Earth these dominants feel it's okay to sit on such a high pedestal. I know there are submissives and DD wives who feel it is their HoH or dominant's right to request anything any time, but I respectfully disagree.

Some dominants and HoHs are of the mind that it makes no difference if their partner is ill, sad, tired, stressed, etc. To me, that equates to being selfish. I care far too much for my wife to force her to do something. We are not infallible, and therefore I need to act as if I am aware of that fact. We are just people, first and foremost. Granted our relationship is structured differently than most, but we are still people who feel, cry, grieve, get sick, make mistakes, and have bad days. To ignore that is to ignore something that is a basic need. This doesn't mean I am lackadaisical in my attitude towards her responsibilities, it means sometimes it's okay to put chores aside if Beauty needs to have some down time.

The point of all this is that you need to think about what or how you view the ideal DD home and relationship should look like.

- Are you standards realistic?
- Will you be able to do all the things you envision in a structured and consistent manner?
- Do your goals reflect what's best for the both of you?
- What is your motivation for wanting to have a DD or CDD relationship?
- Are there any parts of your plan that are selfish?
- Are you honestly able to control yourself if given so much power?

Set realistic goals for yourself and your partner. Establish what will bring punishment and stick to it. A long list of rules is a sure way to set yourself up for failure. Do what you say. Don't threaten, just do it. Instead of becoming annoyed by your partner's failure to do as you ask, avoid the useless and annoying speeches and simply say "Go get the hairbrush." Your authority will diminish if all you do is fuss and threaten. I do this, I admit it, but seriously, if I use the excuse that I'm too tired, it isn't a good one. If I am able to fuss and become boiling mad, then I have enough energy to give a good hard spanking.

Goals, rules, and expectations must be discussed when they are put in place. You simply can't add a rule or punish for something on a whim. Of course things will come up that aren't on the list of agreed upon duties and expectations – for example, your partner doing something that could have resulted in them being hurt. That deserves a good spanking, but in general, keeps to what has been set forth and communicated about. A partner who has no idea what their HOH wants, or gets punished for things not discussed will grow to fear the one in charge. I never want Beauty to fear me. She can have a fear of the hairbrush, but not of me. There will be more on punishment later.

    Make sure you can carry out what your responsibilities will be, and that your partner can realistically carry out the duties set out for them. Learn from mistakes; don't let them rattle you. Everything isn't going to go as planned right from the start, and be accepting of things that you have no control over. When things at work are crazy I am not the calm and collected HoH I like to be. What's important then, is to contain my stress and anger. It isn't Beauty's fault my job is super stressful; therefore she shouldn't bear the brunt of my fury. The same thing applies if my mom gets ill and needs Beauty to help care for her during the day, I can't expect her to get her chores done too. People are human and things crop up that can throw the best laid plans out the window.

    Remember to:

- Govern by example.
- Be firm and fair.
- Be realistic.
- Keep things structured.
- Communicate before adding a new rule or expectation.
- Keep in mind what is best for both of you.

Creating an Outline for My TiH

I have put Beauty's duties and expectations below as well as touching on punishment. This will give you an idea of what a structured plan for your partner might look like. Of course everybody is different, and my expectations and consequences for Beauty will differ from a list you create. I wrote this outline, and then put it before Beauty so we could discuss it together. Some of the things are non-negotiable; some could be tweaked or revised to a certain extent. It is not possible to make a realistic outline that will work seamlessly for both partners without knowing each other's needs. I'm not saying the TiH or submissive should be able to change the things that the Hoh feels are vital, it means that some issues may be amended to best suit all involved.

Loving domestic discipline is an intricate part of my relationship with my wife. Beauty gets punished if she fails to do as she is told. My expectations for her are clear. She is not subjected to discipline at my whim. The reasons for punishment are always well-defined, concise, and understood.

Punishment in our home can be corner time, speech restriction when we go out (Our friends get this. I wouldn't do it in a vanilla setting), or she gets spanked. A punishment spanking is done over my lap, on her bare bottom, with a wooden hairbrush. It is in no way intended to be the good kind of spanking we practice in our BDSM recreational fun. It hurts, badly, and it makes my disapproval known in a big way. It also gets my wife back on track.

Once it is done, she is forgiven, and gets cuddled. When a punishment is over, her indiscretion is over. I do my best not to bring it up again, and she does her best not to break that rule or fail to do her housework again. Let me emphasize again that she has agreed to this, and while she dislikes the punishment, she wants to be in this kind of relationship where I have control, and spankings are part of life. I have her consent to punish her as I see fit.

Many people do maintenance spankings. This is done perhaps weekly, or even daily with some couples. In my home, it is a reminder spanking that isn't done with the hairbrush. It is done by hand or with a leather slapper Beauty likes. Reminder spankings help the person who is the TiH stay on the right course and feel centered. It is an act that creates bonding between the couple, and it helps in keeping things running smoothly. I confess to letting these slide, and I shouldn't. They are very important. I get wrapped up in the stress of my life, and even though I tell you now that I know that maintenance spankings are a great stress relief for us both, fatigue often gets in the way. I need to improve here.

These types of spankings are a valuable part of DD, as is the cuddling and forgiveness afterwards. All spankings in our home are given with love and are done when I am calm. I never punish when I am angry. NEVER. At times I am sorely tempted, I'm only human, but when I punish Beauty, the intent isn't for me to let out my anger, it's to teach her a lesson and get her centered and back on track. I can't do that when I'm mad. I will readdress the subject of punishment in more detail a bit later.

What follows is the outline of expectations, duties, requirements, and consequences for my wife. They are written here exactly as they were presented to her, and were given before we included consequences for negative behavior.

<u>Personal care requirements</u>
- Take all needed meds.
- Get enough rest.
- Body must be free of hair aside from head and small area above bits.
- Nails kept trimmed.
- Wine kept to a two glass maximum and not consumed on a daily basis.
- Eat a well-balanced diet as well as keeping mine well balanced.
- Notify me of any illness, health, or financial concerns immediately.
- Present self as I request, i.e.: Wear maid outfit, lingerie, naked, etc.

You are to reply to direct requests, duty reminders, or reminders about what time it is or that it's getting late with "Okay" or "Yes, thank you" or some such. Not "I know." I remind you in order to keep you on task and to help avoid punishment, so do not respond as if I am nagging. The alternative is to let you just lose track of time without giving any reminders and to take any incurred punishments because of forgetfulness or letting time slip away. The choice is yours, but then you must own the consequences.

Daily

- Household is to be neat and tidy. Clutter is to be at a minimum. Everything needs to have a place and is to be returned to its place after use. This includes dresser tops.

- No TV or computer after 11:00. Reading only.

- Room readied for sleep by 8:00 p.m. This mean bed turned on, water bottle filled, window shades drawn, nightlight on. (I go to bed early because of my work schedule. I don't always require Beauty to come to bed as well.)

- Kitchen counter and floor kept free of spills/crumbs/mess.

- To do list will be kept in mind when planning your day's activities and time you get up.

- Obey all direct orders, including that it's time for bed or to be in bed at a preset time.

- Jot down requests so they are not forgotten.

- Submit to maintenance spankings as they are scheduled.

- Provide sexual release when asked for and or submit to play. I understand tired/sick/etc.

- Relate any misdeeds, concerns, or needs. Weekly conference will be held Saturday evenings. I still expect any misdeeds to be reported as they occur.

- Maintain list of things we need to keep and create a list for bi-weekly Sam's Club shopping trip.

Weekly

- Clean bathrooms (quick clean only. Wipe surfaces down with Clorox cloth or your choice of cleaner).
- Vacuum.
- Change linens on bed.
- Cook a dish that can be used for 2 or 3 meals and cook the special item I request for the week.
- Give me a manicure that may include application of clear polish.
- Clean out refrigerator of unused or old food.
- Empty garbage cans in prep for trash pickup.

Bi-weekly

- Deep cleaning of bathrooms including toilets/floor/mirrors.

- Wash floors.
- Plan dinner menus.
- Dust (including knick knack shelves and blinds).
- Vacuum furniture.

Consequences

Beauty loathes the wooden hairbrush, so other forms of punishment are not often needed. Punishment for not doing daily requirements will be given daily. Punishment for failing to complete weekly tasks will be dealt with on Saturday evenings. If something such as disobeying a direct order, being sassy, or misbehavior occurs during the week it will be taken care of that night. If we are going out on Saturday, punishment will be given before we go. Numbers reflect hairbrush strokes and may include corner time as well.

- Disobedience, breaking rules, sass, or failure to relate misdeeds – 40
- Missed daily tasks – 30
- Missed weekly and bi-weekly tasks – 30

This of course was a working document, that doesn't mean I develop new rules at whim. It means that as we grow as a couple, and as new things come up, punishments have to be tweaked to make them relevant to suit situations that arise.

The Inevitable First Punishment

The first part of this book has been based on things that are important to me and how I handle them. I have covered how I believe the the HoH should conduct themself, the role they play in a domestic discipline relationships, as well as listing some of the behaviors I like to see in my TiH. I've listed what I think needs to be discussed and communicated throughout the relationship, and I've also given you a template of a sample schedule for the TiH as well as listing possible tasks and punishments. These are all things you need to know to start on your journey in establishing a solid domestic discipline relationship, but they have been based on my own personal experiences. The next section will be based on a more general knowledge of things I've learned over time.

As I've noted, each relationship is different. Everything must be discussed prior to instituting a domestic discipline or power exchange relationship. You must define what each partner need and wants, and find a common ground. Clear guidelines have to be established. Even so, with all these things in place, it still won't prepare you for that moment when you realize you must stand by your rules and expectations, and actually punish your partner.

Those into kink won't struggle with this if impact play is part of their dynamic, but those who have never struck the person they love may very well be hit with a feeling of sick dread or a moment of panic. This is when you must remind yourself that both you and your TiH have discussed everything prior to this moment. You have agreed that discipline needs to be a positive factor in your relationship, and therefore it is the HoH's job to carry out the promised consequence.

The HoH may be tempted to discuss the infraction instead of punishing their TiH, but that is the wrong approach to take. A discussion must take place, but it is not a sufficient substitute for disciplinary action, especially if it's the first time a spanking is needed in your new DD relationship. Relax, take time to steady yourself. Get a clear picture in your mind about why the spanking is justified. You need to be settled and confident. Send your TiH to the corner so both of you can reflect on the wrongdoing. Remember, both of you created and agreed upon the code of behavior and chores. Your TiH should know without you having to say a word what she or he has done. If the punishment isn't because of failure to do something on the list of chores or the breaking of a set rule, then you better have a good reason for the spanking. Never punish on a whim.

After you've gotten yourself into a proper mindset, calmly tell your TiH why they are being punished. Yes, I did state that they should already know, but the reason why is always part of the pre punishment lecture. You should also make it clear exactly how they need to act in the future to avoid another punishment, and ask them why they feel they failed to do as instructed. This isn't meant to throw blame on the TiH, it's meant to clearly convey why you are disappointed and feel there is a need for discipline.

The pre punishment talk can be held face to face, that way the TiH must look into the eyes of the HoH and see the disappointment there. This isn't a joyous occasion and the TiH needs to know that. Even those who engage in impact play dislike punishing their partner and your face will reflect your disappointment and regret. The pre punishment talk can also be done when your TiH is already over your lap as you stroke their bottom. They can't see your face, but they can certainly hear your tone, and the stroking is a clear reminder of what is to come. This is one way to smoothly transition from the pre discipline talk into the spanking and lecturing that comes next.

Either of the above approaches can work well, but I tend to favor the face-to-face talk when it's the very first spanking. Most TiH and submissives feel horrible when faced with the disappointment of their HoH or dominant. The disappointment is only part of the reason for eye contact. They must know you won't enjoy paddling them, and seeing their reaction to your words will also tell you if they are indeed sorry for what they have done. Of course they will be sorry after the discipline has been carried out, but you will want them to feel remorse simply because they let you down. Anyone can spank long and hard enough to make someone sorry; it's the feeling of remorse before the punishment that really matters. The painful spanking is the icing on the cake. It reinforces the consequence for bad behavior while also helping to release any guilt the TiH may harbor for their actions. The spanking wipes the slate clean in the minds of both partners.

After the pre spanking talk, be firm, decisive, and in control. Remember, anger has no place in a punishment. If you do feel angry, send your TiH back to the corner. Never wield a hairbrush, paddle or strap when you are mad. Once you feel in complete control of yourself, position your TiH. I prefer over my lap. Yes this is a punishment, but the intent is to strengthen the bond between you by showing your TiH that you care about them enough to correct their bad behavior and choices because they negatively affect your relationship.

Once your TiH is in place, begin with some warm up hand spankings, especially if this is the first spanking you've ever given. These should be hard enough to warm the skin and give it a rosy shade of pink. These aren't meant to really hurt. They are a brief spanking usually given by hand that prepares the nerves in your TiH's bottom for the harder spanking to come. I usually stroke the bottom for a moment after the warm up, and then make sure my arm is wrapped tightly around my wife's waist before beginning her real punishment spanking. Holding her ensures she won't wiggle away and it also gives a feeling of being secure.

Beauty gets spanked with the hairbrush and it doesn't take many to get her kicking and squirming. If you and your TiH are close enough to be involved in a power exchange or DD relationship, then you should be able to read their body language pretty well. Sometimes there is a set number of spanks with the hairbrush and therefore I stick to what was agreed upon, sometimes I paddle good and hard for as long as I deem necessary. Your partner is going to squirm, struggle, cry out, and say ow and ah. It takes someone who is quite used to being spanked to hold still when they are getting a good hard paddling so don't expect this. I do not, however, allow hands to come back in an effort to protect their bottom or to rub it.

When I am done Beauty's bottom is red, not pink. Her tears come more from having to have needed the spanking than from the amount of pain I inflict. I know my wife, and it doesn't take much to make my point. I think with a first spanking you should tread on the lighter side. I am not saying go real easy, but just make your point known and stop. You and your TiH can discuss the spanking later and you can see just how long the redness lasts and if there was any bruising. You will come to know the difference between ow, ow and ahhhhhhhhh. The point isn't to spank and spank until they are a blubbering mess, the point is to spank to ensure your TiH understands that you will stick by your vow to punish and dish out whatever is needed.

Please remember that this is meant as a tool to bring you closer. Cuddle your TiH after the spanking, dry their eyes, stroke their hair, hold them tight and tell them it's all okay again. You are NOT spanking to the point where your TiH is screaming, crying, and begging for mercy. I mean really begging. As I stated before, my wife has a safe word. I don't think she'd use it during a punishment, but she could and I would accept it. To disregard a safe word or clear signs that your TiH has had enough will make them fear you. There is no love or honor in being feared. Beauty obeys not because I have the power to spank, but because she respects me and my authority and believes in me. I have no intention of ever changing that by going overboard in a discipline session. Take it just a little easy the first time around. It is a learning experience for both of you. Honest feedback is needed so any punishment can be effective no matter how hard or soft you deliver the strokes.

The Importance of Bonding, Communication, and Nurturing

I have addressed the importance of seeing to the needs of both partners, how to add structure, and spoken about how imperative it is that both people in the DD or power exchange relationship have the same views in regards to discipline and control. I've also briefly touched on the issue of punishment. There is another area of great importance that should never be left out of any type of relationship, these are the rituals and routines that create bonding and provide nurturing.

The people who are involved in domestic discipline and power exchange relationships will often tell those who question their lifestyle choice that the addition of structure and discipline has brought them much closer. While there will always be naysayers and those who remain skeptical, those of us who live in these types of relationships will undoubtedly insist that it's true. The act of giving guidance, creating structure, holding someone accountable, seeing to their every need including the need for discipline, creates a special bond. There are no long periods of resentment, unresolved anger, or holding on to things that fester and gnaw at a relationship. Issues arise, they are handled in a way that both people find not only acceptable, but desirable, and the problem is laid to rest.

Do DD couples argue? Actually no, we don't. I give her a stern talking to in conjunction with any discipline, but there are no cutting words tossed out while fighting, because fights don't occur. While I fuss when I get weary and she hasn't held up her part of the relationship agreement, I do not belittle her or humiliate her, and I never punish when I am angry.

Beauty can tell me things she feels need discussing, she can give her point of view, but that is all. She has given all the decision making over to me and we simply don't argue. She may say "Yes but..." and I will listen, weigh her thoughts, and then decide, period. Do I ever make the wrong decision? Of course I do, but Beauty knows I did what I thought was best for both of us. I let her wrongs disappear as soon as any needed discipline is over, which most of the time it isn't because she doesn't get punished for mistakes, and when I make the wrong decisions she forgives me after I apologize.

Now some may say that isn't fair. I don't get spanked for bad decisions or the wrongs I commit. I would agree that it wasn't fair if I was making decisions based only on how they would be the most beneficial for me, but I don't. They are honest mistakes, and knowing that I made a bad choice that caused a negative result to happen to my family is a huge punishment for me. It isn't a spanking that makes the hurt physical, but emotionally knowing I screwed up hurts badly. I take my role in the relationship very seriously. I am the provider and protector. Making all the choices when you do so with love, it really pains me when I mess up. I feel as if I let my family down. That's why Beauty doesn't get disciplined for making mistakes. We all make them, and she makes far less of them because she has my guiding hand in all she does. The weight of worry is lifted from her shoulders.

Domestic Discipline isn't some kind of nirvana for those who give up control, but it does give the TiH a sense of peace because the major worries are my worries. Nothing can take away every single worry and bit of stress from anyone's existence, but the structure and discipline DD relationships hinge on makes life easier for my wife and I. I do battle with the big stressors, and she fights all the little everyday battles that get on my every last nerve. I know I don't have to worry about the prescriptions being picked up, the pets being taken to the vet, gas put in the car, or what's for dinner. It's all done.

One analogy I like to make, when trying to explain that Beauty does indeed like her role, is to equate it to what really made us feel stable and safe as kids. When we were children, it was the adults who cared enough to hold us accountable for our actions and gave us structure that made the biggest difference in our lives. As adults the same rings true. I am in no way equating a domestic discipline relationship with a relationship between a parent and child, but even when we were kids, we knew which people in our lives really made a difference even if their choices for us were unpopular. We all thought the kids who were allowed to do anything they wanted were the ones to envy, but being allowed to rush headlong into bad decisions sets people up to fail no matter what age they are, and so is allowing someone to think the world is all about them. It is those people who never learn from their mistakes, hurt others (including their families) by being selfish, and never grasp the importance of responsibility. Some of us thrive on being given structure and correction, and some of us thrive on providing it. Each role comes with responsibilities that help to give us self-worth.

To have self-esteem is one of the basic things we need in life for happiness. That saying about how you must love yourself before anyone else can love you is true, and DD relationships help foster self-respect. Many people don't really understand the whole appeal of being submissive. How it can be a positive thing can be hard to grasp. There is much talk in the kink community about the gift of submission. Some like to use that term while others will roll their eyes or scoff. Whether Beauty's submission is a gift is really irrelevant. The thing that matters is the fact that Beauty trusts me enough to hand over total control of her life to me. You can call it whatever you want, but what it comes down to is a huge affirmation of trust. That show of trust binds us. It gives us both a feeling of being important to each other, but that trust had to be earned.

I doubt many people would develop a sense of trust for someone who said one thing and did another, or a person who seemed to punish them harshly or with glee. When I discipline my wife it certainly doesn't make me feel happy. The fact is that even though I enjoy impact play, I only discipline Beauty in instances where it must be done. There isn't pleasure to be had and she knows it. Punishment is a somber thing in our home. It is done because I love her and she needs correction to keep her life in balance. It is because of the fact that I find no joy in spanking her as a means of discipline, and only punish her when it is justified, that she has given me her trust.

My wife knows I always have her best interest in the forefront of my mind when I make decisions. She knows that when I take the hairbrush to her bottom it's because I care enough to correct her and to help her live up to her potential. She also knows that once she has been punished the slate is wiped clean. Being completely forgiven and having the wrong made right with a painful spanking that releases any pent up emotions or frustrations, and then being cuddled as I stroke her hair, both of us knowing the issue is done with, is freeing. I feel so much love for her as we cuddle, her nuzzling into my chest, my arms wrapped tightly around her. The naysayers can have their doubts; I know that it makes our marriage stronger.

One of the things that bring our relationship closer is maintenance spankings. The time spent with her curled in my lap with a well warmed bottom creates a bond. I take the time to snuggle with her, to hug her and give small touches. These little shows of affection let Beauty know what she does is appreciated, as does saying thank you and meaning it.

I also make certain there is time set aside each week for us to sit down with the expressed purpose of speaking freely about any concerns either of us has. I set a schedule that makes certain she gets enough rest as well as one that provides time for her to relax with an activity she enjoys every day. All of these things nurture Beauty and our relationship. They show her I value her and care if she is happy. The intent of our relationship is about nurturing the body and the heart. Discipline is never given with the intent of belittling her.

If you wish to have a DD relationship you must be prepared to punish with specific and loving intent. Always make it clear why your partner is receiving the chastisement. If you can't verbalize the why of it, then perhaps the punishment isn't justified. Your actions must have clear purpose. Don't let the power of your position of dominant or HoH go to your head. You are not more important than your submissive or TiH.

If you have a sadistic side, then find a masochist for a life mate or a play partner (this can be and often is nonsexual) for BDSM play. Do not use an overly heavy hand when giving a punishment. That isn't what punishment is about. Punishment isn't fun, it doesn't give either partner pleasure, but used correctly, it can help create a relationship that is rock solid. One where the TiH feels secure, and one where the HoH is confident, compassionate, loving, and fair.

Find time for each other every day. Don't take your submissive or TiH for granted. Listen to each other and have respect for each other's needs. Don't be demanding, and don't be spiteful. None of those things are beneficial to any relationship. It is the dominant's job to keep their partner grounded. When a punishment is over, let it go. Only revisit the misdeed if it occurs again. If things aren't running smoothly, look to yourself first. Your partner follows your lead. Never forget that power can be a double edged sword that must be wielded with care. The success of any DD or power exchange relationship rests on the shoulders of the dominant and their ability to be ethical, just, compassionate, and loving.

Pitfalls, Disillusionment, Burnout, and Mistakes

Every book you pick up on domestic discipline talks about how the HoH needs to stay in charge and discipline the TiH when needed without fail, but I haven't run across too many articles or books that focus on what should happen when the dominant screws up. Before I go into specifics as to what makes a quality dominant and how yes, we too screw up, I want to speak on the signs of or characteristics present in those who are not being a good dominant.

This first section of this chapter is geared towards the submissives and TiH, and addresses things they should be on the watch out for, because there simply are things a submissive shouldn't accept. That being said, the dominant or Hoh should read this as well, because if you see yourself in any of the points that follow, you need to examine your actions.

If you are a submissive or someone who wishes to be a TiH, please read the next section carefully. If any of the following points holds true for someone you meet who thinks of themselves as a dominant, turn the other way. These things go beyond the natural differences in domination styles. I am a huge nurturer, but a person can be a good dominant without being a nurturer just like I can be a good dominant without following the more rigid principles. There are things however that should never be accepted.

Someone is not a good dominant if:

- They think it's all about them.
- They demand respect or being addressed by a respectful title before you are their submissive.
- They do things without your consent to test you or to make you prove you really want to be a good sub.
- They ignore your limits or tell you that you shouldn't have any.
- They try to cut their TiH, submissive/slave off from their family and friends.
- They are emotionally abusive and make their s type feel vulnerable, ashamed, weak, or not a valued person.
- They think the s type should take care of them and that's it, no give and take.
- They ignore your safe word or say you can't have one.

It is imperative to listen to your intuition whether you are considering a new relationship or involved in a long term one. If it feels wrong, it most likely is. If it hurts in a bad way, get out. No matter your role, TiH, submissive, or slave, you have a right to leave, and you don't have to do it alone. The Leather Heart Foundation which can be found at http://www.leatherheart.org or on Fetlife.com can help you, even if leaving means you would be alone without any money. This unfortunately can be a pitfall when giving the power of everything in your life to someone else. Often times you have no money of your own or have no control over the finances. You have a long span of years where you weren't employed, and you possibly have lost contact with some family and friends because of your lifestyle choice. A good dominant takes care of their partner until they are on their feet, but this isn't always the case. Be informed and make smart decisions when choosing a dominant. Don't be impatient and don't let your need for discipline and structure blind you. Take your time, ask questions, and get to know a prospective dominant before agreeing to anything.

To be a good dominant you have to be willing to work hard to fill your submissive partner's needs. To find a good dominant you need to seek someone out who is interested in the real you, not a puppet or a blow up doll, or a doormat. Submission is a gift, but so is good dominance. Look at the person outside of the DD or BDSM box. Yes that stuff matters, but there is a person in there too.

Now for the pitfalls. It takes a great amount of energy to be a proper HoH. You have someone depending on you to take care of their needs. I am guilty of not remaining consistent, keeping control of myself, and letting Beauty slide on a punishment because I am tired at the end of a work day and don't want to have to deal with her failure to carry out a task or some other misbehavior. Instead, I fuss at her. We've been married three years now and I have at times dove head first into the pitfall of losing consistency.

I let the fact that I am tired stop me from having her fetch the hairbrush and bend over the nearest chair.

Sometimes I tell myself it's because I am too angry to administer a fair punishment, sometimes I am so stressed I truly don't have the energy. The truth of the matter is that if I carried out a swift, short, and effective spanking then and there, I'd save myself a lot of fuss and stewing about her lack of following her schedule. The energy spent being upset far outweighs the energy spend using the hairbrush on her bottom.

Being tired is no excuse for complacency. If my wife is failing to do as she has been directed then I need to address the matter in the way we have agreed upon, give her the discipline she has earned, and be done with it, knowing she will do as expected the next day. I know this, I see the positive outcome of a good spanking, and yet I stumble into the "I'm tired" pitfall too much. It is important to watch for this and to avoid any fussing and frustration that will be caused by the lack of a proper response to her misdeed.

Another pitfall is not looking at the big picture when things aren't running smoothly. Again, dominants should look at their own actions and what's going on in their lives rather than focusing on the lack of actions of the submissive or TiH. There are things that interrupt even the smoothest running DD relationship. We were recently in a car accident, followed by my 87 year old mother needing emergency heart surgery. The two events were unrelated but they created havoc with our lives and our schedule. My serene household wasn't so serene. There were a million phone calls to make, runs to the hospital, working with insurance people. It all made for a couple of crazy months.

I will be brave and say there were days I fussed at Beauty about the state of the house or the lack of something I needed, but I wasn't being fair. Her plate was overloaded and I never punished her for the fact that my place of serenity was a mess. Inside I knew she was doing her best. My anger at the chaos made me shout at her, and in effect made me lose that control a dominant is always supposed to display. I admit it and am not proud of it, but I tell you of it in this book because the pitfall of having tunnel vision and expecting the things around you to remain tranquil and unchanged crops up in any relationship. Look at the big picture and adjust your submissive's or TiH's schedule so your expectations are on the same level of his or her abilities in the face of something unexpected causing turmoil.

The next issue that can muddy the waters of any DD or power exchange relationship is what to do when the dominant becomes weak. It is inevitable in any long term relationship that the person who is the HoH or dominant will become ill and unable to carry out the role they normally play. I'm not speaking of being sick with a cold or the flu; I'm talking about a serious debilitating injury or medical issue, something that makes the dominant feel like they have lost power. The important word there is feels.

We experienced this in my marriage when I began having seizures that mimicked a stroke. I was weak, had a very difficult time speaking, and had to rely on Beauty to walk. It left me feeling as if I was powerless because my body wasn't working. I felt as if I was unable to carry out my role as HoH. I felt that the structure I usually created and the guidance and discipline that was meant to be provided was out of reach because we had to focus on me and my needs. Being physically weak made me feel like I was letting my family down even though Beauty never added to those negative emotions. They came solely from me.

The pitfall here is one the dominant actually falls into, not the submissive or TiH. One might believe that without the usual power evident in the relationship supplied by the dominant that the TiH would flounder, take advantage of the lack of discipline, or not be able to shoulder all of the responsibilities, but that doesn't turn out to be the problem. The problem is with the feeling of uselessness the dominant feels. The complete lack of power and control is something the dominant almost fears. They worry and many don't want their submissive or TiH to see them when they are weak. I know of a few dominants who actually tried to push their submissive away because they couldn't put on a strong front, but I learned that it didn't matter if I was strong or not. My teachings and the dynamic of our relationship was strong enough to weather my time of extreme weakness because our life and the things I taught Beauty stayed in place even though I was weak as a baby.

Beauty lay next to me in my hospital bed. She brought things from home that I might possibly need, she stayed with me all through the nights and took care of me for the months that followed as the doctors got the seizures under control with medication. There was no need for me to be strong, but it gave me a hard knock on my psyche anyway. I didn't have the strength to do any chest thumping and say "I am dominant hear me roar", and I didn't need to. Beauty carried on with things as usual even when those things meant caring for me like I was used to caring for her. It didn't make our dynamic come to a grinding halt, it actually made Beauty thrive. She didn't flounder without my direction, instead she was well prepared to face whatever came our way head on. She had the rock solid foundation we'd built together.

Beauty is a caregiver at heart, and she returned all the nurturing I had given her. We weathered the storm without my strength because the very nature of our relationship enabled my wife to be strong enough for the both of us. That period of our lives together prove to the naysayers that a strong DD relationship is healthy and benefits both partners. Me making all the decisions and setting forth what she should do every day for most of our relationship didn't leave Beauty unable to carry on when I was sick, it left her able to thrive in her role of caregiver, and we both found that she had the skills to take on all aspects of our life without missing a beat. I struggled to accept my weakness, but finally came to terms with it, and I marveled and was so very proud of my wife as she took the reins while I recovered.

So the moral of the story here is, don't feel as if your submissive or TiH shouldn't see you when you are weak. It's okay if something leaves you unable to be strong. If your relationship is well rounded and healthy, your partner will be able to care for you and take on the job of running the household, so do not push them away. Her respect for me remained, our dynamic didn't change. She didn't run free and misbehave; and she most certainly didn't take advantage of my weakness. Instead she used the strength I had given her and carried on as usual.

Almost any issue that comes up in your relationship can be resolved with honest communication. As I said before, make a certain time each week for the two of you to sit down uninterrupted and talk. At first this may feel awkward but don't give up on it and decide to forget about it. Be persistent. Maybe some weeks you won't have much to say, or just maybe your partner will tell you of some deep seated worry or fear. Just talk to each other. Dominants need to use this opportunity to share as well. Are you feeling burned out? Is there something your partner is doing repeatedly despite correction that needs to be discussed and analyzed? Don't fall into the trap of getting angry and fussing or shouting, do what needs to be done and get the paddle or hairbrush. It takes less energy to give a spanking than it does to stew over a misbehavior or lack of completion of chores.

Talk, carry through with the discipline you have put into place when things go off track, and remember to always look to yourself first. It could very well be the dominant's lack of follow through that is causing the problem. The blame game helps no one. Find the cause of any trouble and take it on, be it a new action on the dominant's part or a swifter means of discipline for the TiH.

How to Punish Ethically and Effectively

The next section of this book deals with types of punishment and ways to punish. It is intended for both those who are developing a DD relationship as well as those in power exchange types in BDSM. Not all of the punishments will appeal to or seem proper to those centered on domestic discipline without any type of kink factor, but it is my hope that everyone will find something useful. I could have placed this portion further down in the purely BDSM section, but the question is often asked of me, so here it is for all to read. If portions offend you, skim over them, but remember that the ethics apply in whatever type of relationship you develop where punishment is a part of it.

When it comes to punishment, there are as many different views on it as there are ways to do it. Many dominants say they do not punish. If a submissive or slave cannot chose to be respectful and show their desire to submit by following the rules set out for them, then they are not interested in a relationship with them. Many dominants feel you shouldn't have to punish an adult. Many, on the other hand like me feel that punishment is a tool to help guide and give structure and limits to one's partner.

I would never become involved with someone who constantly tried to break the limits I set and expect to be followed. I don't have the desire, energy, or time for that nonsense. Brats never appealed to me. My wish was to spend my life with someone who wanted the structure and the discipline that a domestic discipline relationship provides. I found that person in my wife. While she hates the hairbrush, she understands that I punish to keep her centered and to help her focus her energy in the right places. My punishments are given with love and never done when I am angry. They help to bind us together because I care enough to call her on her misbehavior and to do something about it. Often times, misbehavior has a root cause in something that is troubling her, and a sound spanking and the cuddling afterwards help relieve whatever stress she was carrying around.

    If you are new and are struggling with a submissive or partner who refuses orders, then the chemistry is probably not right. My wife is a pretty good example of this. She was a brat, plain and simple, so I did not pursue a D/s relationship with her though we were both very attracted to each other. I did not give her the dominance she craved inside until she decided that she truly wanted that type of relationship. I laid things out for her and told her this is what I expect. I didn't battle the brat, I let her need for a D/s relationship override her rebellious attitude and sass. She was and is very well behaved. Our friends could not believe it when I said she was good, but she was and is. It just takes the right approach and know-how.

    In a new relationship or one you are thinking about starting, set the bar high, but keep it reachable. Lay out your expectations and stick to them. Do not go into a relationship thinking you can change this and that. Yes, working on issues your submissive or partner has through behavior modification is okay and often done, but that isn't what I'm speaking of. I'm saying if a person you have interest in refuses to obey or they aren't ready and willing, they will simply be a huge headache. In vanilla relationships, as well as in D/s ones, you shouldn't start out thinking that if you can change X,Y, and Z, they will be a perfect match.

Now I will list punishments I have done for the breaking of rules or not doing as told. Again, this is the occasional mistake or disobedience, not methods I use to break a submissive. I don't break people; I have no desire for that annoyance. These all must be done with communication. Even ignoring should be discussed so the submissive knows exactly why they are being punished. Also, when a punishment is over, I let the infraction go. Taking the punishment is like wiping the slate clean.

- Ignoring - This is the absolute worst punishment that can be done for most submissives. New submissives may want to push you into a punishment that they desire. The best way to nip this in the bud is ignoring them.

- Corner Time - This can be done with or without a spanking. Most submissives dislike corner time. In a sense it is like ignoring. I do not speak to my wife when she is in the corner, though I am not truly ignoring her because she is where I can see her. Again this can be a "Go to the corner to wait for your spanking." This is good if you are feeling anger. Do not physically punish your submissive when you are angry. Or corner time may be used after a spanking. The submissive must go to the corner to think about what they did and stand there, often sniveling, with their punished bottom on display.

- Speech Restriction - After my wife had back surgery I could not spank her for a good long while. She did not do as told when packing for a trip to a kink event. She loves to visit with people we haven't seen in a long time but because of her behavior I put her on speech restriction for the first evening when we went down to the dungeon. Simply said, she could not speak a word. She put a card that said speech restriction in her plastic thing that held her badge so people knew why she wasn't talking. This was a hard punishment for her. She did very well and I relented about half way into the night. This is a good punishment for masochists. You can't give them physical punishment because they like it so it isn't effective.

- Loss of Playtime - My play partner (completely non-sexual) gets told if he doesn't behave he won't get beat. Now I am kidding 99% of the time. He isn't my submissive so I don't punish him. He is a huge, huge masochist so any physical interaction is enjoyable but NOT playing would be a truly bad punishment.

- Spanking - I have a wooden hairbrush that is reserved for spanking. We never play with it. Beauty hates the thing. It stings like hell. Having an implement that is reserved only for punishment can be effective. Physical punishment doesn't have to be spanking. Let me state here that I do not believe a hard limit should be used as a punishment. Something your submissive/slave dislikes but has consented to is okay. Maybe they dislike flogging or canes, so you flog or cane them, but again, this is if they are NOT a hard limit. Also, unlike 'funishment' spanking or erotic spanking, I do not bring Beauty to orgasm after a punishment spanking. I do however hold her close.

- Difficult Chore - My service guys do as they are asked for the most part. Only once have I disciplined one of them, but in the case of a submissive doing a sloppy job or not doing as asked, then some menial chore such as the old scrubbing/cleaning the bathroom floor or toilet with a toothbrush can be effective.

- Many guys have a fantasy about doing a menial task dressed as a French maid or other feminine outfit watched over by a mistress dressed in the stereotypical dominatrix outfit holding a crop. If this is the case, take yourself out of the equation. This kind of goes back to number one. If a submissive failed in doing a job correctly, I would simply show them where I found the task lacking, tell them to do it again or in case of punishment, tell them the specifics, then go sit in the living room until they were done. I would not allow feminine clothing. The whole scenario would be reserved for a reward. Don't punish with something a submissive enjoys.

- Using rice creatively - Some have a submissive kneel on rice for a given period of time, some spill rice or some other small bitlets and have the submissive pick up each and every grain with a tweezers. Again, there would be no element of me standing over the submissive dressed in black leather holding a crop for a punishment.

- Intended painful anal sex - Again, let me stress that if something is a hard limit you do not use it for punishment. We had a huge conversation on the board about a guy whose submissive had anal as a hard limit because she was raped in that way and he used it to punish her. This is a huge NO! Painful anal must be done carefully. You do not wish to do physical harm. If a sub dislikes anal but has not put a limit on it, or if they like it but only with a lot of prep so the pain is almost nil, then this is an effective punishment.

- Anal punishment and anal sex – **You must have consent from your partner to include anal chastisement as a form of punishment when the dominant or HoH feels it is warranted. If you use anal sex to punish without consent, you are committing rape**.

    Both anal punishment and anal sex are very primal. The one on the receiving end really feels submissive. You **must** prep your partner to the extent where there will not be tearing or physical harm. You can use lube and use your fingers or a small plug to stretch your partner beforehand. Taking someone anally is a very dominant action in and of itself. Go ahead and punish anally, put a dildo in while you are spanking, or take your submissive anally and harshly, but do it safely and use lube. Using spit is gross and is only done in porn movies. **Use lube, don't take a chance of causing internal tearing, and have consent! Non consensual anal sex is rape. Rape is not punishment, it is a crime.**

- Public humiliation - This can be in the form of forced feminization, wearing a sign that calls one out on their behavior, posting on the board that they have been bad and telling of their wrong. Please note that anything that can be considered kinky should only be done in a BDSM gathering. Forcing your submissive to be on a leash or dress as a woman, etc. in vanilla public is forcing your kink on the vanillas and is not okay.

- Denial of orgasm or forced orgasm – I have done both with a submissive who has masturbated without permission. You can set the time of denial for as long as you know your submissive will suffer because of it. Often you can add bringing them to the edge then stopping. Again, the time period can be a day or weeks, depending on your submissive.

    Forced orgasm can be very effective too. If a submissive has been touching herself without permission I will use the Hitachi to make her orgasm over and over until she begs to stop. You do need to be careful here. The Hitachi really causes intense orgasms. If you make her cum over and over watch for signs that her body really can't take anymore. My wife can get headaches if she cums too long and too hard. You can always take a break of a few minutes then go back and do a few more forced orgasms, then take a break etc. I normally will take a strap to my submissive's hands and fingers as well if they have been touching without permission.

- Pussy punishment - It is no secret that we are super sensitive here. I usually will give pleasurable sensation first so the clit is enlarged and then use a leather strap/paddle implement I have to spank or punish the pussy. You can add a hard fucking of the sore pussy after strapping or spanking it. I tend to only add fucking if we are playing and a rough sex scene is wanted.

Be creative. The best punishment is something that your submissive dislikes and gets your point across without breaking limits. You need to know your submissive to find what they dislike but are okay with. I will not be goaded into a punishment. I will not punish in anger. I will not give punishments repeatedly. Punishment must be done in conjunction with conversation. I always tell Beauty why and have her tell me why she is being punished. Repeated physical punishments without talking about the why of it are useless. Many dominants do not punish, they simply talk about the infraction and state why it wasn't okay. Again, if a submissive continues to misbehave then really, most of us would cut them loose. In an established relationship this would be a sign you really need to communicate, in a relationship that is just starting, it would be grounds for dismissal.

I laid out my rules and expectations and we talked about each of them, and then Beauty agreed. She knows what will bring punishment. Often times simply knowing I am disappointed in her is enough. This is where communication comes in. There is no tossing in new rules, testing her loyalty by making her do things she has as a hard limit to prove herself worthy, or a constant change in how I expect her to behave. TiH, submissives, and slaves need consistency and structure. If your submissive is misbehaving, then as a dominant, look to your own actions as to why they are not living up to agreed expectations. There is usually a reason why someone continually does not do as told. Communicate, communicate, communicate.

Keeping a Domestic Discipline Relationship Free of Abuse

 People who aren't into a kinky lifestyle or who don't understand the intricacies of domestic discipline may easily confuse it with an abusive relationship. It's vital to make the distinction between an abusive relationship and DD or D/s one. I encourage Beauty to have outside interests, to be creative, to do things she enjoys. I allow her speak freely to friends and family and in no way ever try to keep her from them. She is allowed to go out alone to meet friends. I trust her; I want her to be happy. She has been trained and knows what I expect of her whether I am with her or not. She doesn't exceed her boundaries and that is out of respect for me and our relationship, not out of fear of punishment.
 On Fetlife.com we ask dominants to address me first if they wish to contact my wife. This is just how we do things. It cuts down on the idiotic emails filled with sexual requests from random guys. She is owned, collared, and married, and therefore I have a say in all she does, but she has a say too. As I said before, she has the right to speak her mind and is encouraged to. I make the final decisions, though. With this power comes the full and complete responsibility for her. I must take care of her and keep her happiness and welfare in mind in all I do. As for the physical punishment, my wife has a safeword. Would she use it during punishment? No, I don't think so, but she could. I would never punish her to the point of her safeword. I punish, I don't abuse and I have no wish for

my wife to fear me. There are those who do not permit safewords, and many a slave and submissive who say they don't want one. Everyone runs their relationship differently.

Our DD home is not a rigid household where she serves me and isn't allowed to speak or must sit on the floor or other strict rules. My wife is my partner, not a lesser part of our relationship. We relax and have pretty normal lives. Like BDSM power exchange relationships, domestic discipline isn't some vastly different kind of mysterious relationship, or at least it isn't most of the time. We are a basic married couple who live day-to-day, often mundane lives. Our recreation is different in the form of BDSM play and friends who are kinky, and the structure of our relationship has a hierarchy to it and consequences for bad choices and failure to obey. That said though, we are just like a 'normal' married couple in most everything else. Many DD or power exchange relationships are like this, especially if they are long lasting, but unfortunately, many are not.

I always check the data for my blog. How many visitors, what did they click on, were there any comments left, and last but assuredly not least, what search terms or engines brought visitors to my blog? I have seen a disturbing trend as of late. Quite often there are searches wanting info on using forced sex to punish your wife or forced taking of her painfully hard for domestic discipline punishment. I have to take a deep breath to control my dismay and tramp down the anger I feel when I see these in the search box. Forced sex is wrong. It is always wrong to force sex upon someone who has not given their consent, period.

Now I know that many are probably wondering about where the line is drawn in a domestic discipline household, and why are some forms of punishment okay, and some aren't. I think it's a fine line those who are in power as head of the household must walk. They have the wellbeing of their wife or partner in their hands and so must tread carefully. One thing I ask myself is 'How will this punishment help the situation? Domestic discipline is really behavioral modification 101, but we are dealing with people here, people we love, not rats or dogs (I am not advocating hurting dogs!). A punishment should be a learning experience, clear expectation should be conveyed to the one being punished, and communication is a must. Yes a punishment is an aversion tactic, but creating aversion does not equal causing trauma.

One of the things I told Beauty when we first became a couple was that she always had the right to say no to sex, BDSM play, or even a punishment, BUT the no to the punishment was only a short reprieve and only granted if she is ill or if I can see she isn't in the right frame of mind to learn something from the punishment. I have zero interest in causing mental/ emotional harm to my wife. Discipline helps us grow and helps us stay on track. She agreed to life in a domestic discipline household before we were married and I collared her.

Some may argue that if a person gives their consent for the head of the household (the HoH) to discipline them, then forced sex should indeed be okay. In my mind it is not. Punishment and forced sex just aren't the same thing. Punishment equals behavior modification; forced sex equals a violation of the body. Forced sex is rape whether it is in a DD household, date rape, or stranger rape. Please do not confuse this with nonconsensual consent BDSM play. That is a whole different thing and it is done by those who like to play rape or abduction or rough/forced sex. This is NOT done to punish. Both parties have given consent.

Like I said, there is a fine line here that those in charge must walk. One thing that is key, is that things have been discussed and agreed upon when the relationship began. That doesn't mean every punishment must be run by the one needing discipline before you can punish, that means you have talked, know their possible trauma triggers, know what is very abhorrent to them, know what frightens them, etc.

Let me try to draw a line here:
- **Okay** – Spanking your wife with a paddle or spoon or hand. **Not okay** – Whipping her with a belt **IF** you know her father beat her with a belt as a child and it can cause terrible memories and flashbacks that could include doing emotional/mental harm. The belt or strap is fine for punishment as long as there is no connection to past trauma. The point is, if it can do harm mentally or emotionally then the punishment is not okay. Find something else.
- **Okay** – Putting a clothes pin on a sassy tongue or instituting speech restriction for

sass. **Not okay** – Pushing your wife's head underwater when she talks back knowing full well she has a horrid fear of having her head under water. This comparison is a bit extreme but I'm trying to make a point. I also know someone who did the not okay example. Shudders!
- **Okay** - Inserting a butt plug prior to spanking knowing full well your wife hates the butt plug and dislikes anything in her bottom. **Not okay -** *Taking/raping her anally or using anything in her bottom when you know that she was once raped in that fashion or has some other experience that would make using this kind of punishment a traumatic experience.*
- I frown on my wife using her safeword during punishment, but on the same note, I don't want her to be biting her tongue to stop from screaming 'red' because I have gone way over the line.

Forced sex is rape unless it is acting out in a BDSM scene and has been discussed as something both parties want. Now you may say "Hey, if she said okay for me to use anything to discipline her that I see fit and she has no prior trauma then why isn't forced sex on the okay list?" Then let me ask, do you really want your significant other to equate having sex with you to be a punishment and really bad experience? Punishment is to correct and once it is done your bond is still in place and the relationship is stronger. Forced sex or raping your wife may be fun for you and may make you feel all kinds of dominant, but does it really teach? Will she want to cuddle in your arms when the punishment is over and her wrongs have been erased or will she feel violated and scared?

People searched for strapping her pussy then raping her. I would say no to this as well unless there are strong elements of BDSM in your relationship and not just DD and, a huge no still to the raping. Some play hard at 'funishment'. They strap or spank the genitals then have consensual sex. That is a whole other thing. Some might fuss and say a slave or submissive cannot say no to sex. That is all well and good. That is the nature of some D/s relationships, BUT I would expect the dominant in this kind of relationship to have compassion for the slave or submissive as a person. Failure to do a chore or talking back does not merit holding one down and forcing painful brutal sex on them.

I don't want my wife to equate sex as something negative. I would not force sex on her to hurt her as a punishment. Why would I want to make her feel unvalued and used? Forced sex (including anal sex) used as a punishment equals rape and it is not okay. Those in charge have the authority to rule their home as they see fit, but they also have the responsibility to protect and nurture their significant other. Rape is not protecting and it sure as hell isn't nurturing.

- Never punish in anger.
- Never punish in a way that will do harm to the heart and spirit.
- Punish with love and compassion.

My wife isn't meant to like a punishment, but it shouldn't cause emotional trauma. I have no wish to have Beauty fear me. Fear doesn't foster respect, fear does not foster love.

The following section is a tutorial on anal sex. There is a safe and pleasurable way to have this type of sex. ***There is also a way to safely use anal penetration as a punishment if your partner has consented to this type of punishment***.

Do not cross the line here. Domestic discipline is meant to be a loving, structured, nurturing, relationship entered into by two consenting adults.

The Different BDSM, DD, and Power Exchange Roles

The roles or positions people assume in DD, power exchange, or kink relationships have many titles and at times subtle nuances. I have done my best to provide an 'average' persona or some characteristics of each of the various roles people adopt.

- **Dominant** – This can be a person of either gender who assumes the role of being in charge. They are the one who makes decisions. They have the position of power and they take on the responsibility of the person who chooses to submit to them. Other dominant titles are:
- **Master/Mistress** – Some women prefer Master. I myself prefer Mistress. A person who identifies as a dominant. One who owns a slave or submissive. That does not mean I am everyone's mistress. I am simply a person in my kink community. I am mistress to only a select few.
- **HoH** – Head of Household in a domestic discipline relationship. This person can be male or female. I am a female HoH in our home.
- **Domme or Domina** – A female dominant.
- **Pro Domme** – A woman who works as a dominant to provide the service of domination for clients. This does not include sex but does include domination in many

forms. Impact play, role play, submissive servitude, humiliation play, etc.
- **Top** – The person who is in control of a BDSM play scene. The one who ties, binds, does impact or sensation, interrogation, etc. The Top and the bottom are not in a power exchange relationship. Their roles are used during the play scene and the aftercare session.
- **Switch** – A person who identifies as both a submissive and a dominant depending on who they are interacting with. Some people do it during play as they enjoy being a top and a bottom depending on what manner of play is going on, some go back or forth in a relationship depending on who they are with. For example, I know of women who are submissive to men but dominant to women. The reverse of this is popular as well.
- **Taken in Hand** - The TiH is the submissive partner in a domestic discipline relationship.
- **Slave** – A person who gives total and complete ownership of themselves to a dominant person. My wife has given me control but she is still her own person and maintains free will through a safeword, open conversation, and sharing her opinions. Slaves can have stricter rules, be on higher protocol such as not sitting on the furniture, not speaking, doing anything their Master or mistress says without question. A slave's role

is completely decided by their Master or Mistress. A slave can be any gender.
- **Submissive** – The person in a power exchange relationship who has given control to their partner. Submissives generally have less strict rules, perhaps are only submissive in the bedroom, have more input into their relationship guidelines, and can be of either gender.
- **Bottom** – A person who is on the receiving end of a BDSM scene. They freely negotiate prior to play and are not submissive to the Top who is directing the scene except for during play. I am fully dominant in all my relationships but I will bottom for electric, violet wand, or neon wand play. It is possible to enjoy being flogged, canned, etc. and still be dominant. Being a bottom doesn't make you submissive, but you are placing your trust in another's hands for a while.
- **Kinkster** – A person who is kinky, or enjoys fetishes and may attend BDSM social munches. They may or may not be in a relationship. My wife is a submissive, TiH in our home but she is only submissive to me, and really identifies as a kinkster in our kink community. She is also learning to co-top with me during play.

There are other roles including those in age play, pony and puppy play, and an ever increasing vast amount of terms with which people identify. I am in no way disregarding any of them, but am refraining from including those that are not part of what I am trying to educate people about with this book.

So You Think You Want to Be a Dominant

I look at the search terms people put in to see what topics appear most often. It helps me keep my finger on the pulse of my readers. Lately, along with the search for information about domestic discipline, I am seeing the desire to find information about having a sexually submissive wife/slave on a 24/7 basis. The search terms are somewhat varied, but they all center on having someone to be a sexual toy at their beck and call. One who follows every order, does all the home tasks, and submits to punishment to satisfy their need to be sadistic or dominating, and is basically a Stepford wife for the one seeking the power. If you are unfamiliar with the term Stepford wife, it comes from a movie where all of the wives in a perfect little upscale community became robotic, perfect wives, obeying every command and fulfilling every desire. This desire, seen over and over, needs to be addressed, because real life and fantasy do not always go hand in hand.

I have news for all those seeking to control a submissive or slave. Dominance takes work. It isn't all about you when you are someone's dominant, and no matter what, unless you are dealing with a blow up doll, you are not going to have an "always ready for sex, never talks back or questions your authority, never expresses their opinion, never has needs you don't wish to fulfill, submissive" or slave. Regardless if someone is a slave or submissive, they are people, and people are living beings that have needs, brains, emotions, and reactions to what happens around them. People get sick, people must grieve for a lost loved one, and people must tend to the vanilla side of their lives. No one is perfect and available at every moment no matter if you are strict, demanding, unyielding, all powerful, god like, or even truly wonderful. No one is perfect, including you.

1. Being a dominant is a double edged sword, and both sides can cut. When you are a dominant to someone you get to make the rules, make the decisions, and decide how your submissive/slave, home, relationship, is going to be run. You are the one in power and yes, that can feel good. I personally am an A type who likes to structure my life as I want it to be. I choose how things are done. I make the rules. I have the power to decide everything, **but**, being the one in power 24/7 takes work and let me tell you, there are times when my wife or my guys look to me for decisions when I just want to have a break and wish they could do things without looking to me for direction.

If you want to control all they do, be prepared to make every decision even if you are tired or not feeling like it. If you want to be in power 24/7, it is going to flow into your vanilla lives and there are going to be times you don't want to have to make decisions or punish, or be in charge, but guess what? You decided you wanted it so here it is. There isn't an off switch on your sub/slave and they will struggle if you are not consistent and don't meet their needs. I feel it's best to empower my wife by allowing her to express her opinions, and my wife certainly has a brain, but she is wired for submission in our relationship and to please me, so that means I am in charge… all the time.

2. If you punish or use other techniques to make sure they all obey, be prepared to never have a vacation from decision making. Where will we go? What will we wear? How should we act? Do I want her to buy A or B? We need a new vacuum. The sink is clogged. Please tell me what to pack. Please tell me what is on the to-do list.

I hope I am making my point here. You get to tell everyone what to do and have things your way, but 24/7 means ALL the time. Many submissives and slaves have taken that role partly because they do not want to have to make decisions or be responsible for the running of their lives. That's their thing. Structuring your world is yours if you are dominant, but be prepared. If you create a person who looks to you for everything and obeys your wishes and commands, you are in charge. No vacation for you.

3. It isn't all about you. – Do not think you want to be a dominant because then you will have someone to do everything for you from

housework to sex slave and everything in between. Wow, is life easy. My slave does all the work. I get to be lazy and play god. Nope. If you become a dominant you become responsible for your submissive or slave. Beauty is my responsibility. I must make sure she is healthy, well fed, has her needs met both physically and emotionally. Receives praise and guidance. Has structure and nurturing. Is disciplined in a way that teaches her and brings us closer, you get the idea.

She gives, she does the housework, she does the shopping, I can say I want to play or have sex, or be driven here or there, or anything that comes to mind, BUT I also must take care of her every need as well as plan for her future. It is my job to make sure she is happy and will be okay financially if I am gone. She is mine 100% and in return I am responsible for her well-being in her submission. It isn't just about me, dominance and submission are a two way street. You can create a relationship where you are only dominant and submissive in the bedroom, or only when you choose to be top and bottom for each other and not have so much responsibility for each other, but what I am addressing is the constant search and desire for 24/7 sex slave and sex slave wife, etc that I see all the time. If you want all the power, then take all the responsibility.

4. Training isn't easy. – Real life is not the Story of O. Yes there are maybe a couple of places in the US that do training, but that just isn't the reality for 99.9% of D/s relationships. So you want a sex slave? Poof, here one is. How will you meet their needs so they always desire to serve you? How will you enforce your rules while at the same time making sure the punishment is meaningful if rules are broken? What is your step-by-step method of guiding and teaching them? How will you help them to learn your ways? How will you care for them when you aren't fucking, playing with, or using them?

A slave or submissive is a live person and can't just be put on the shelf or into a toy box. What if they are ill? What if they need extra love and compassion because they are in menopause, grieving for a parent, or are bipolar, or whatever need that isn't mentioned in the porno BDSM movie on training a sex slave?

5. Are they content in their servitude? Are they getting fulfillment from being your slave? They want to be a slave because it meets an intrinsic need; are you doing what was agreed upon when you entered the power exchange relationship? Very few slaves or submissives just want to be chained up and ignored unless they are being used. We all have vanilla needs. Any slave or

submissive needs to be taught how you want things done. It can't just be expected and you can't just tell them a long list of rules. People make mistakes. How will you deal with them? Better yet, how will you deal with yours?

6. Punishment isn't meant to be fun so don't expect it to be!!!! - I have explained the difference between punishment and 'funishment' before but I'll say it again. Punishment is something that is disliked by the submissive/slave. It is a negative happening in response to their breaking a rule or being disrespectful. I do not like to punish. It means I must do something negative to my wife. Before I punish I must look at WHY she failed to do something. Was it a lack of communication or simple defiance on her part? Why and how can I make sure it doesn't happen again? It isn't she was bad or didn't obey so now I get to spank her and fuck her in the ass to show my displeasure and get my kinky desires met.

7. My rules on punishment have been stated before but bear repeating.
a. I never punish in anger. I will never hurt my wife when I am mad. I must be calm and in control. Send her to the corner or whatnot until I am calm.
b. I always make sure my wife knows why she is being punished.
c. I talk to her and communicate with her

during the punishment.
d. I strive to make it a learning experience.
e. I forgive her when it's done, show her love, and take steps to make certain she will not repeat her infraction.

Funishment is play punishment. Funishment is fun for BOTH of you. Your sub/slave should at least get something out of it. If you love anal and your sub/slave doesn't, go ahead if it's not a hard limit but make sure they receive praise for serving their dominant and make sure you do anal safely. If it is a hard limit do not go there! Being a dominant doesn't mean you get everything you can dream of. Your slave/sub should enjoy 'funishment' and be taken care of during and after it.

If you are a sadist your sub/slave should be a masochist to some extent. My wife is not a huge masochist but I can find fulfillment in our play. Just because I do not flog, whip, paddle her until she is black and blue and full of welts, I enjoy our play because I get the same reaction from her to my toned down play as I get from my super sadistic play with my play partner who can take anything I dish out. Yes, you can push your sub/slave. Yes, you can give them a dose of something that stretches their limits; yes you can design a scene around your pleasure, but it needs to have something in it for them and it needs to have aftercare.

- If you love humiliation don't choose a sub/slave that does not thrive or like it.
- If you are a sadist, don't choose a sub/slave who hates pain.
- If you are turned off by a man wanting to cross dress, don't take on a sub/slave who lives to wear women's panties and loves to be made to do chores in frilly things.
- If your sub is service oriented, then allow them to serve. Don't expect heavy sadistic play.
- If you love needle play do not take on a sub/slave who is frightened of needles and has that as a hard limit.
- If you are a nurturing type of dominant don't take on a sub/slave who is a huge
- Masochist and doesn't like to cuddle.

You should have things in common from the start, both in the kink world and the vanilla world. Always remember, **Punishment = a negative consequence** that a sub/slave can learn from. A way for them to know they have done wrong and to be told or shown how they can do better. It is not enjoyable. **Funishment = an enjoyable BDSM** scene where both parties get their needs met.

All you "forced anal punishment" people listen up! Forced anal is bad, it is <u>rape</u>. Forced anal 'funishment' can be scripted in a scene so it hurts some, so it plays out like heavy force, so it makes you feel as if you are taking her or him by force. BUT, have consent and be mindful of your partner's needs. It's not all about you, and as I state in my anal tutorial later in this book, if you take steps so they like anal sex you will get more anal sex without ever resorting to rape.

Anal sex whether it's a 'funishment' by force scene or straight up kinky anal sex should satisfy both partners in some way. It's okay if you like anal and he/she doesn't. You have the power to say yep, we're doing anal as long as it isn't a hard limit. Just remember it isn't all about you. If you do anal on someone who doesn't care for it, make sure the scene gives them pleasure in some way. That can be said for any 'funishment'. Think about and care about your submissive/slave/play partner.

Never forget reality verses fantasy. So, you want a slave who is chained up naked unless you feel like using her? Reality – Depending on where you live, clothing or blankets are a reality and no one should be made to sit chained all the time. Yes, some wish that in a scene or in part of their life, but the 'always' is not a reality. They have to eat, sleep, use the toilet, exercise their bodies, have human interaction, receive praise, and receive some kind of positive interaction from their dominant/get their needs met. This doesn't mean you have to be all cuddly if that isn't your dynamic, but if being nurturing hasn't been left out by mutual agreement, then you need to provide it.

As stated, a slave is a person. Maybe they want to be in a cage, maybe they want to be used as a table, maybe they want to be treated like an object or humiliated, but you can rarely do these things 24/7. Whatever it is you think you want in your sub/slave, you had better make sure they are okay and their needs are met. Even those in cages need to be let out for exercise, tables get sore knees and need to move about, humiliation should be desired or else you are simply being emotionally abusive.

Anything done simply for your own pleasure needs to have a positive outcome for your sub/slave. They are human, they have needs, and they came into the relationship looking for something. Are you making sure they are getting that something? People have to get up, get dressed, go to the doctor, go to work, visit with vanilla family, and take care of the vanilla side of their lives. That is reality.

If you want to be a dominant then you had better be up to taking care of another person. If you want a slave then you better be up for REALLY taking of another person. You can't train someone to be a slave, to never make decisions, to never leave the house without you, to never speak, to never do one tiny little thing you don't approve of and then drop them because you get angry or bored. Having a slave means you will care for them as they get acclimated back into society if things go wrong. You will be there until they can stand on their own two feet mentally, financially, and physically. Having a sub/slave means you see to their needs along with yours. If you think it's a game, find a partner who only wants to play occasionally, don't try to take on the responsibility of a 24/7 slave.

- Punish responsibly.
- Have compassion.

- Be able to take on the responsibility for another person.
- Dominate with caring or love.
- Don't be egotistical. It isn't all about you.
- Be creative.
- Accept fault in your sub/slave and in yourself.

Being a dominant is a job! Do it responsibly or don't do it at all.

You Think You are Submissive. Now What?

Much of this book has been devoted to the HoH or dominant in a relationship and how they should go about creating a strong and stable environment. I have repeatedly addressed the need to include the TiH or submissive in the negotiation and process of drafting a document that will work for both partners, but I haven't said much on the subject of being submissive.

This first misconception I want to dispel is that a submissive person is weak. That simply isn't true. It's more about the role in life they wish to live than a lack of qualities that make some people appear strong. It takes courage to give yourself over to another and vow to do as they say. Refraining from making decisions can lift a weight from one's shoulders, but at the same time it can cause much anguish if the one who is submissive feels at all unsure of their chosen dominant's ability to rule with respect and fairness.

Many a submissive person has sat alone after reading an erotic tale of submission or coming upon photos or blogs on the internet. They identify with the submissive character of the book and think that is how they want to be or to live. There is a huge gap, however, between doing and dreaming, and that is where it becomes hard to navigate the waters.

There are dominants who are really just bullies who prey on those who are submissive. That isn't just an opinion. There were times when I was discovering my kinky dominant side that I had a rough time of it. After the loss of my first long term submissive, I ventured into the world of online kinky personals. There was ALT and Collarme along with some others that didn't cater to those who were kinky. I soon found that both are riddled with imposters, emotional sadists, and in general people who were there to get their kinks.

My wife was first brought into the world of dominance and kinky play with the Anne Rice Beauty Series. It opened her eyes and sparked a desire to not just be spanked, but to be controlled and have oh so naughty things done to her. She tried to steer her husbands in that direction, and then navigated the twisted arena of Alt and Collarme too. Neither her efforts with her husbands nor the websites brought her any success.

Once single again, she made the choice to get out into the kink community. A new submissive woman in the kink community, despite there being many upstanding dominants and submissives, is like tossing fresh meat to the lions. I am in no way trying to paint a bad picture of the kink community. I am a big part of ours, and have many great friends who are not only ethical, but wise. It's just that when a new submissive woman comes into contact with a group of male dominants, they tend to act like kids who want a new toy. Though many have the best intentions, when someone is new, they need time to make friends, learn, have a chance to talk to people from all sides of the spectrum, and make careful decisions based on choices made over time.

There is an article on sub frenzy on my blog that is worth reading, because it is a phenomenon that affects many submissives. My advice to those who are new is to find a submissive person to be your guide or mentor. Do not choose a dominant for this role. A protector should listen to and guide you. A protector should call you on your bad choices. They should be someone you respect enough to actually listen to their point of view. A protector should never be someone you engage in BDSM play with, and the relationship should be platonic. A good protector should know those in the community. They should be able to steer you to someone who can safely teach you about rope, impact, sensation, or most any other type of play you think you might be interested in and would like to try.

A person you want to experience something with does not have to be your dominant. You are giving them control of the BDSM scene while it's taking place, but you keep your control by participating in the negotiation held before hand, during play by having a safeword, and afterwards when you say thank you and walk away. A close submissive friend or mentor can help with that final phase because you may be floaty and in sub space and not able to make good decisions at that time. You may very well feel a strong attachment to the person you had a scene with, but please make relationship choices later.

While you are learning AND waiting to meet the right dominant or person who could be the perfect HoH, please remember the following:

- **Stranger danger** - Seriously, as a submissive you are vulnerable, especially after playing. Don't go out to someone's car or home with them. Choose a partner who is well known and respected in the community.

- **Have set limits –** These can change over time, but know your limits and share them right away. During any play you might say ok to things that are not. Limits can change as you learn. Limits should not be changed during a scene. Where is it NOT okay to be touched? What is your stance on bruising? What are your expectations for aftercare?
- **Listen to your intuition –** Is there something that feels wrong? Do others seem to avoid the person? Are they trying to get you alone to play instead of playing in the public play space or a friend's home? Do they say they don't believe in safe words? Do they brag about all the things they've done instead of taking time to get to know you?
- **Stay off Craig's list!**!! – ALT and Collarme are bad, but running off to meet someone from Craig's list is dangerous.
- **Be diligent –** When I was searching for a partner and using websites, I developed a system to try and screen out the off balanced and posers. Always try for verification. Remember, webcams can record now so anything you do for someone might end up on YouTube. I used to have people take a photo of themselves holding a current newspaper or a sign with the date on it. This can be falsified, but can help.
- **Be patient –** Don't jump in head first in person or online. The right person will come

along. Before meeting in person at a SAFE place have at least three chat sessions. Most people can't keep their cover for long if they are hiding something. In person meetings should be done with a safe call. Let the person you are meeting know you have a safe call and set a specific time you are going to call your person. Don't leave your safe call until you get home safe. Set a time to call during the meeting and stick to it. It's also a good idea to have a safe phrase. That can be something like "I was going to wear the red dress". A phrase your safe call is listening for that means everything is really okay. It may sound like overkill, but it keeps your head out of the clouds AND keeps you a bit more grounded. There is no such thing as too many safeguards when you are getting to know a potential dominant.

- **Develop yourself** – Be smart, learn about how other's live power exchange relationships and domestic discipline relationships. Learn about yourself and what matters to you. Don't compromise the things that are important. You can learn and experience without latching on to someone who is questionable.
- **Be strong and have pride in yourself** – You are not weak. You have the right to be respected. You have the right to ask any questions you want. Those who tell you a

submissive should never question a dominant are either full of themselves or hiding something. Any dominant is not YOUR dominant until you are in a relationship and therefore demanding to be called Sir or Ma'am and telling you questions are rude should be scratched off a list of potential dominants.

- **Being submissive doesn't mean submissive to everyone!**
- **Submissive doesn't mean less than a dominant.** It is a give and take relationship, one where you are vitally important.
- **Be smart, stay active, make friends** – Fetlife.com is pretty much a Facebook for those of us who are kinky. It is not a meat market like the other sites though you will get hit upon. The fact that you can't do a mass search for submissive women makes it harder for predators to find new prey. Fetlife.com offers over a hundred groups to join and learn from. The one for submissive women is a great place to start. You can ask questions, read from the shadows, pore over the groups of kinks that interest you. There are ones on Domestic Discipline as well as ones for Slaves and Masters. It is a place to learn and make friends as well as to find local get togethers.

Remember you are your own person. Don't let someone treat you badly. An experienced submissive of the same gender should always be at the top of your friends list. They can teach you about the ins and outs better than anyone, but avoid those who try to draw you into play by saying their master or dominant wants to add a third to their dynamic. Just find friends. There are also ethical dominants out there who will help you learn. Just take your time and stay aware.

The Power Exchange of Service Submission

There are many types of power exchange and D/s relationships. They take on many forms and are best done through a combination of compatibility, needs, fetishes, kinks, and expectations. Without communication a relationship won't be a good fit. Toss out your misconceptions, take a good look at your own needs, and how much time, work, and emotion you are willing to take with anyone who wishes to submit to or dominate you.

One area of power exchange that has a lot of misconceptions is that surrounding the relationship of Mistress/Master and service submissive. There are those who will say that a true service sub doesn't exist and those who will say that no matter what, the dominant is taking advantage of the person who wishes to simply serve and receive nothing in return. I wish to dispel those ideas. The true service submissive does indeed exist, and I am in no way taking advantage to the men who serve me.

The interviews, discussions, trainings, are all very detailed. Everything is laid on the table beforehand. Both sides come to understand what the other is seeking. While it's true that I met with and interviewed a good handful of men who really weren't service submissives, I also found a few gems who are. They are wonderful and have become part of our kink family. We have grown close over the last few years, lines that were drawn have fluctuated just a bit, there has been light play added on a very rare occasion, but basically they come, they do the list of (as one of my guys prefers), "man chores", they visit, they receive hugs and thank yous, and they go on their way.

They want nothing but appreciation, and I make certain they get it. We value them and they care about us. There is no wearing of the maid outfit or frilly outfits while I stand over them with a crop as they work. That isn't the arrangement that was agreed upon. Our first guy wore his ladies underwear under his clothes but that was it. He came over to do chores. Hang things, clean, cook dinner to give Beauty a night off, fix a bad faucet, clean the car, you name it. Adam has run free now and no longer serves us, but he and we had a great relationship.

We now have two other men who serve us. One for the yard, and one for most anything else. They both serve at parties but are given a chance to play with any guests. I help with negotiation, make sure they are safe and get aftercare if they play, but with Beauty and I, they simply serve. Dick loves to be here. He arrives with a smile, does his chores with efficiency, and follows directions - be they written or verbal - with ease. He doesn't need supervision. He wants to be here and leaves with regret that he can't stay longer or do more.

What I'm getting at here is that yes, service submissives exist. I know because I have them, and it's not because I am lazy. Beauty needs help at times, I am not skilled in fixing things like Dick is, we have a need of his expertise, and he has a need of service. Our house has the variety of things go wrong that houses do, and Dick knows how to make it work again. From plumbing, to carpentry, to electrical fixtures, our home would be lacking without Dick's help. He wants no money, no BDSM play, no fetish fulfillment unless service is a fetish. He wanted to experience impact play so we had a short session because he is always so deserving but the fact is, he doesn't want more. So that's my message here. Yes, they do exist, but they are hard to find. It all comes down to matching needs and personalities. Communication is the big factor here.

    In the next section I have outlined part of my interview procedures that any service submissive of mine must fill out. We go over it in detail. The fetish list is there because I want to know what they might be seeking, or so that if they do wish to experience something, I can find them a safe and sane partner to play with. It is made clear from the start that our roles in the power exchange will be Mistress and service submissive. This type of relationship may not be the thing for you, but I am including it so those who are interested have the information, and because it is a form of a power exchange relationship. If nothing else, perhaps it will help those who wish to outline questions for a domestic discipline partner, a submissive or a slave. Remember, learning is the key, even if something isn't for you, having knowledge about it makes you wiser.

Pre Service Checklist and Rules Prior to Becoming My Submissive

These are the things I give to and go over with, my service submissive guys prior to them becoming part of our kink family. We discuss it, go over each point carefully to make certain they understand each one completely. I then make certain through communication that they agree to the rules and consequences. My rules and requirements for Beauty are much different and have evolved as our relationship went from just beginning to long term, to lifetime marriage and collaring. These rules and expectations are only partially fluid. Everyone, no matter the type of power exchange relationship they're in, has things in life that change who they are and what they are capable of giving to another person.

I have maintained the questions and checklist as they are given.

Pre service/play checklist

You are to complete the following checklist. If there is something you have done check it and follow the check with L for liked, D for disliked, N for not sure. It if is something you want to try, mark it with a T. If there is something you have no interest in, simply put no. If it is a hard limit put H. You may leave something blank. Also, just because it is on this list does not mean I do it so do not answer in an effort to please me. Put question mark if you don't know what it is. {The format of my list is a bit different, but you get the idea.}

anal plugs	lingerie	high heels	breath play	role play	shoes	high protocol
age play	knife play	cross dressing	slapping	cling wrap	fetish events	electrical play
humiliation	speech restriction	erotic literature	crawling	discipline	orgasm control	kneeling
spanking	sexual service	vacuum bed	collar and leash	cages	fire play	exhibitionism
flogging	chastity	cupping	vibrators	whips	switching	stockings
objectification	bondage	CBT	prostrate massage	masturbation	submission	voyeurism
water sports	suspension	foot worship	strap-ons	forced masturbation	TPE	anal sex

List any type of kink that you are interested in that is not on the list.

_____
_____
_____

List any health issues or limitations I should be aware of.

_____
_____
_____
_____

List any fears (these will **not** be used against you to torment you. I need to know so I do not trigger an unintended emotional trauma).

_____
_____

What image or idea sexually stimulates you the most?

_____

Fill this out to the best of your ability. Mail one back to me via email, make a copy for yourself and bring it with you when we meet for your interview.

These are a bit redundant but there are a couple of different ones.

Rules:
These are iron clad and must be obeyed. Failure will result in punishment. Punishment may include but is not limited to: Spanking, corner time, written apology, public declaration of misbehavior (on Fetlife), denial of orgasm, loss of privileges. Repeated or deliberate breaking of rules will result in a loss of trust.

Note to my readers: I would never give a spanking to someone who is deliberately attempting to misbehave in order to receive one. I am too wise for that, and someone who would do that wouldn't pass all the pre service interviews anyway. If a spanking or punishment is needed for anything, it will be something they do not enjoy.

- What happens in our D/s family is a private matter. This does not mean you may not ask questions of others/mentor. Just do not disclose private family information.
- Do not disobey a direct order.
- Never arrive for service intoxicated.
- Share any health concerns or issues that affect your service immediately.
- I share these now so you know what I will not bend on. Expectations, ways of service, rewards, etc. will be discussed.

This is another document that is gone over prior to service and entering into a service agreement and power exchange relationship.

Expectations:

- You will always address us with a respectful title. Yes Miss, No Miss, May I please Miss, Miss would you like? Thank you Miss, etc.
- All tasks are to be done to the best of your ability, taking heed of how you have been told or taught to do it. For example: If I ask you to dust, you will carefully put things back in their place, and if I were to check for dust anywhere when you were done, I would find none. You will indicate you are done by saying you have completed all your chores and would I please inspect your work.
- Privacy is to be maintained at all times. What you observe/hear in our home and things done with us stays among us. Your privacy will be respected as well. Discretion when arriving at our apartment and leaving is a must.
- You will ALWAYS phone when you have to cancel an appointment or are going to be late. Be warned, I am not patient when it comes to tardiness unless there is a very good reason. Repeated cancelling of appointments will result in my feeling as if you are not committed to being my submissive.
- You will not serve any other Mistress or engage in play with another while serving me. If as you become more acclimated to the BDSM lifestyle and

you are more interested in trying new things, tell me. I will make arrangements to accommodate your interest IF you have earned it.
- You will obey Miss Beauty as you would me. If you are in doubt about an order from her, do as she has told you and ask me about it later.

Possible Tasks – Your duties will include but are not limited to:

- Household chores – You may dress as you wish for this, once you have earned the privilege. If you prefer something frilly that will be acceptable. Your chastity device must always be worn. Failure to do your chores correctly will result in the loss of privilege to wear frilly outfits.
- Foot massage, manicures, pedicures – I suggest you read up and watch some YouTube clips on proper manicure/pedicure techniques. Miss Beauty cuts my nails. You would shape them, apply polish, and finish with a massage. Miss Beauty will be pampered with this as well. Back massages will be included as well once we are all comfortable.
- Cooking and serving a meal to us. This of course includes clean up as well.
- Hauling groceries, heavy chores Beauty cannot do alone. Tasks that are handyman type. Butler type service at play parties.
- Accompanying us to events. This is for munches and dinners as well as private play parties and big events. You would be expected to come with us if

your schedule allowed. You would get drinks, open doors; make sure we had what we needed. At events you would carry suitcases, load and unload the car, put away clothing and arrange shoes and fetish outfits. All dates and times will be discussed. I am not unreasonable and do understand real world obligations.

- Serving at dinner parties.
- Wash/gas up/vacuum the car.
- Simple secretarial duties such as making phone calls, answering emails, etc.

Rewards:

- Praise from your Mistresses.
- Orgasm if they are to be denied for any length of time.
- Directed masturbation.
- Expanding your duties so you know we are pleased with your work.
- Permission to use a butt plug when serving. Inserted by you.
- Flogging sessions.

Consequences:

It is always best to ask for clarification. Asking will not bring a reprimand unless it is something that has been asked about repeatedly. Not doing something properly, or failing to perform up to my expectations, will result in you being disciplined. When you are disciplined you will always be told why. It will not happen on a whim. It will not be done in anger, and you will always be told what must be done to correct the problem.

Discipline will consist of:
- Hair brush spanking.
- Corner time.
- Loss of masturbation privilege.
- Public posting on Fetlife that you failed to please your Mistress.
- Cancellation of a future fun event/playtime.

Punishment spankings will be administered to your tolerance level. If you are being punished it will hurt as it is meant to so you learn your lesson, but I will take into consideration that you have not experienced much of this and I will adjust the number you receive. Your safeword is respected during a punishment spanking but it is frowned upon. Punishment does not = a serious beating. A spanking would consist of 10 to 20 swats. More swats if it is an offense that has been repeatedly committed or if it is a rule that has been broken. Paddling and corner time or public post can be combined.

Questions:

- How do you feel about serving at events?
- Do you understand about a safeword being respected during punishment but frowned upon?
- What are you most nervous about entering into this venture?

- What handyman skills do you possess? Do you have skills such as woodworking?
- Can you cook?
- Do you understand what level of protocol I expect at all times?

How to Approach a Mistress

I received the following email on my Fetlife account awhile back, (my Fetlife name is Inaralee) and I have to say I get a lot of these even though my profile states I am married, monogamous, and not seeking a submissive. I wanted to share the email in an attempt to educate some of the submissive males who read my blog. This is not meant as an attack, just basically a WTF, and a "Please pay attention to what I am saying." to increase your chances of finding a Mistress.

hi,
I am new to this lifestyle, when my gf tied me up and played mistress i was introduced to this world, at that fraction of time i realized what i want in life.
I am a sub male looking for a mistress who wanna own me for 24×7. I'm a very submissive guy! Can tolerate any amount of pain inflicted on me by my Mistress, All I need is my Mistress pleasure and satisfaction! I live to please her I love being humiliated and punished! I can survive on this my whole life! I want to get collared and made a dog of my mistress I just wanna be under the divine feets of my Mistress serving her
regards, sub

- I don't know a single dominant woman who would respond in a positive nature to someone who lives as far away as this man does from me. There are women who do online, but unless they indicate that is what they are seeking, being far away is an issue.

I really do not for the life of me understand how someone can be of service if they cannot come to my home live and in person.

- I NEVER ever, consider a guy for a submissive position who I wouldn't meet live in person at a munch two or more times when I am surrounded by my friends so I know he is not a creeper. The guys who are my service subs are people my friends know, and ones who I have met in social settings. No one comes to my home until I am very comfortable with them and am sure they are safe. I take my role as protector of my wife seriously. If I don't know you well and my friends don't know you well, you never get asked to my home. Seriously, that is the stuff of crime shows and Lifetime movies.

- If you want a mistress to consider you, open with an email telling about yourself, not telling what she can do to you. Add something that shows you read her profile and offer something that would be enjoyable for her as far as service goes. The above email is very clear that he didn't read the part that males only have the role of service submissive in any relationship other than friendship. I don't care about the other stuff. He didn't say anything that spoke of an effort to read my profile or let me know why he thinks he could serve me, not some fantasy Mistress. Mistresses are women first. Dominant people second. Appeal to both and speak of vanilla interests that you have in common.

- Do your best not to come off as a do me sub. That is someone who says either I like this and I like that, or do this to me and do that to me. Remember, the objective is to SERVE her. Oh, and skip the 'You can do anything' stuff. I mean really? I can roll you in honey and put you on a nest of fire ants? No one sane says they will do 'anything' to someone they don't know and have not established trust with.

- If a woman is seeking a male submissive for a long-term or possible lifetime relationship, again, appeal to the woman and the mistress in her. Romance goes far as does conversation outside of the BDSM and sexual talk.

- I met all of my guys in person face to face at munches. Munches are not events where play takes place. They are just get togethers at a bar or a restaurant where kinky people get together to talk and socialize. If you really want to meet dominant women, get out and get active in your kink community. A guy my friends know and trust and who I have met has a much, much better chance of ever being in service to me than a guy who sends an email. Actually the email guy has zero chance unless he is local and willing to put in the effort of getting to know me a bunch of times at local munches.

- The above man states that his girlfriend tied him up and played mistress and he knew in that fraction of time that he wanted to be a no limits 24×7 submissive. For one, real mistresses don't play mistress, it's part of who I am, and it is impossible to know that you wish to live out your life as a 24×7 submissive simply from being tied up. My message here is know yourself, I mean really know yourself by reading, talking to, and interacting with people to educate yourself and discover what you really want in your role in BDSM. We are starting to come out of the closet, people, and the wealth of serious information is everywhere. Still, meeting with people who actually do BDSM and live in power exchange relationships are the best way to learn and try things safely.

Again, this is an attempt to educate, not berate the guy who sent the email and other guys out there that are searching for a dominant woman. Be yourself, be real, treat her like a person, be respectful but not a doormat, and don't live halfway around the world.

How to Approach a Submissive and the Idea of the Submissive Slut

Many men who are first becoming enthralled with the whole BDSM thing are under the misconception that if they become a dominant or toss out orders, they will then be able to have their pick of women who will fuck and suck them and say "Yes Master" to any of their desires. This twisted view of the submissive woman annoys me to no end and so I am going to provide my views on submissive women and sexual promiscuity. I'm going to pull out my soap box now so I may say things you disagree with but as with all my advice, your mileage may vary.

To avoid sparking anger, I want to make it clear that I am not speaking of all men when I speak of the middle aged, horny men who exhibit through words or deeds the degradation of submissive women. I am speaking of those who really have no clue about BDSM and what a healthy D/s relationship should look like. Most of these guys pick up their knowledge of kink by watching bad BDSM porn or reading stories to jack off by on the internet. They think hey, I can go online and find a woman or even go out to a munch and be all Domly by ordering some young sweet thing to do as I say and we'll both be happy. Woo hoo, I have found the secret to getting laid! The reason for this misconception does originate in the porn out there so there really isn't any blame in it. I am not throwing mud at the clueless, but I am slinging it at those who have been told and should know better.

Heads up, people... submissive does not equal slut.

Submissive women do not go around following orders from men they do not know and drop to their knees to suck someone off because they were told to, and what's more, no woman is a whore, slut, nasty bitch, etc. outside of her own relationship. It is NOT okay to use those terms with a submissive woman unless she is yours by mutual agreement and it is part of your play and relationship roles. My wife can be my dirty little slut, but I better not ever hear anyone else call her that. I would never use that term in public, aside from in a public dungeon where most of those present are busy playing and know that she is MY slut and mine alone. The "mine" there refers to both the physical as well as someone else simply using the term.

Slut, whore, cunt, nasty bitch are often used as terms of endearment in D/s relationships. You see paddles and collars with those words on them. They are used as acceptable terms and often are almost akin to a pet name. Some use them all the time, some, like me, use them only during sex or play. If I call my wife a slut during play, you'd better bet that it doesn't mean she sleeps around. Talking dirty is foreplay and often people do 'funishment' that includes the submissive being punished for being wet, for becoming aroused by a spanking, or for being a whore with a fictitious partner. If I call my wife a whore and get rough with her for it, it will get both of us aroused. If a stranger calls my wife a whore or expects services because she is submissive, they will be flayed alive verbally and possibly hit. Try touching her because you think she is easy because she is kinky, and you will most definitely be hit.

I will say it again: Submissive does not mean easy. Seriously, submissive does not equal being a slut. If you walk up to a submissive woman at a munch or even try to be dominant and order a woman around because that worked for a guy in some book or porno, you will possibly be slapped and most definitely won't get laid.

Submissive women deserve respect. So do submissive guys, but that is a whole other area and deserves its own chapter. Treat a submissive woman like you would treat any vanilla woman when you first meet, and for god sakes don't send crude emails on Fetlife or Collarme or wherever with dick pics and crude comments. That will NOT score you any points. If you would not say something or want something said to your sister, wife, daughter, then refrain from saying it to a woman just because she identifies as submissive. "Do me, bitch" is not a good pick-up line. Submissive women are not waiting all eager and ready to spread their legs for any strange man who tells them to, so stop thinking and acting like they are.

Now for another issue under the same topic. Having multiple play partners does not make a woman a slut; in fact, I would advise someone who is new to meet people in the community and find out who is respected and who is known to play safe in order to learn more about themselves and different fetishes. BDSM play does not have to be sexual. It is intimate because there has to be a trust and communication bond between the players, but that doesn't mean playing with different men is being a whore. If someone is new and wants to try bondage, then they should seek out a trusted community member and try bondage in a public place/dungeon to see if yes, it is good. If someone has a fantasy involving spanking or paddling, then yes, find someone who is trusted and does safe impact play and try it out. If you are turned on by whips, or anal play or even being bound to the cross and having your clothes cut off, then find a trusted member of the community who does safe kidnap and knife play and try it out. The point here is that doing and learning with someone safe does not make a submissive or bottom and slut. It is literally just playing. BDSM play, which is pretty much like recreation for those of us into kink, doesn't mean we all run around having orgies and gang fucking some nubile submissive woman on the pool table while she cries 'Oh please, fuck me harder'.

I have multiple play partners and I am not a whore. My play with my wife is sexual, my play with my other partners is caring and intimate, but it is not sexual. At our last play party someone had a Sawzall which can be altered by the use of an attachment, to make it a fucking machine that pistons forward, and back at a fast and steady rate. My wife wanted to try it and I certainly was not going to take the thing and use it on her because I had no knowledge of the tool and how to use it safely.

I spoke to our friend who had brought it and we set it up so Beauty could try it. She was essentially penetrated by this man using a dildo and a power tool, but it was a play session. Did she orgasm? Yes, but it was play, not sex. There was more intimacy between she and I because I was on the floor next to her holding her while she was being penetrated. Our friend who was using the Sawzall on her was not part of the intimacy between us. The same would go for fire cupping or cutting which I have little knowledge of. If she wanted to try those things I would find someone who knew what they were doing, and negotiate a play session. Play does not mean sexual intimacy. It means the kind of stuff we do for recreation.

1. Submissive does not mean easy or promiscuous.

2. If a woman is called a slut, whore, tramp, etc. by their dominant, it is not an invitation for you to do the same.

3. Submissive women and men deserve respect. They are just people and should be treated with normal, socially expected courtesies.

4. Having multiple BDSM play partners does not equate having a sexual relationship with all of them, or make one deserving of the term slut.

5. My calling Beauty a slut is okay, someone else calling her that or sending her letters that say 'do me' or whatever is rude and insulting.

6. Use the manners your mother taught you when dealing with women involved in BDSM. No one is your whore or your submissive

until you are in mutual agreement of that fact.

7. And one last thing for the record. It isn't okay to call a woman a slut or treat her in a degrading manner even if she does have multiple sexual partners. Some people enjoy lots of sex with different partners, some prefer to be monogamous. No one deserves the title of whore or slut.

Anal Sex Tutorial/ How to introduce Anal Sex

I have decided to add this section on how to safely introduce anal sex into your relationship because the interest in anal sex is the number one topic people search for. I am also somewhat dismayed because people find my blog by putting forced anal sex or anal sex as punishment in domestic discipline in the search engine. If you are a HoH or dominant that thinks forced anal sex is a good way to discipline, please read the section about forced anal sex used as a punishment either in a domestic discipline situation or in a D/s relationship.

In that section on discipline, I say that in no way is it acceptable without complete consent. I will say it again. Forced sex is rape. Please, people, there are plenty of women and men who love anal, and a lot who have never had it done properly that would like it if they had a good experience with it. If you find pleasure in being the fuckee while engaging in anal sex or really want to try it and wish your wife, girlfriend, or boyfriend was open to trying it or allowing you to boink them anally, then proceed properly and introduce them to a pleasurable new sexual act.

Anal is not for everyone, and those who say 'no way' should be respected. If you get consent, then please follow the steps below. Do not think it's okay to hold your partner down and fuck them anally. That will destroy any hope you ever had of getting them to give consent in the future as well as making them afraid of or resentful of you.

What you need ahead of time:

- Towels and anti-bacterial wipes - Anal sex can be messy both because of the lube and because mess can happen. I always have issues getting the lube off my hands after I use my fingers to play with and open my partner's anus to relax them and when I lube up the dildo. Anti-bacterial wipes are good too, but putting a towel down is a good idea as well. Remember your fingers, dildo, or cock will still have bad bacteria on them if they are not washed or you have used anti-bacterial wipes. Wiping your hands off on a towel makes them less messy, but not clean enough for the mouth or vagina.

- Lube - I like Liquid Silk. Lots of lube will help make the experience good for both of you. Seriously, the stories of guys, or women with strap-ons, shoving their cock in using only spit for lube is a bad idea. I also think that even when wet with your partner's juices, the anus needs lube before pushing in. You can cause tearing inside the rectum that can lead to a bad infection and serious health conditions. A tear in the rectum plus poo full of bacteria is a disaster waiting to happen. IMO just say no. It's a bad idea.

Prepare your partner ahead of time. They will want to make sure they are cleaned out. Enemas work well for this. You don't need the whole enema bag kit unless you both are into that. A Fleet Enema kit works fine. Please be respectful and allow your partner privacy if they wish it. Things having to do with the butt can be embarrassing. Yes, I know that humiliation can be a kink, but make sure it's consensual. Give your partner sometime after the enema so they aren't feeling like they still have to go. If this is your partner's first time they need to know that despite every effort to be clean inside, mess can happen. Putting a condom on your penis or dildo is a good idea.

Once your partner is clean, lay them on the bed on their stomach on a mound of pillows, bent over on the spanking bench, or over your lap so they are feeling comfortable. Remember this experience is to be enjoyable so they will be open to doing it again. Make sure towels and anti-bacterial wipes as well as lube are close by. Use your fingers to tease their anus, rub your lubed finger over it and round and round, getting them relaxed. Don't just go and shove your finger in. The key is subtle play: tease, circle, rub until your partner is noticeably relaxed and even moving with your finger or indicating they want more. Fingernails must be trimmed or cut short and clean. Remember, you don't want to tear the inner walls.

Start slow, just the fingertip in with very gentle in and out movement. Make sure your finger is well lubed. Get more if needed. There really is no such thing as too much. Well, the whole bottle is too much, but use your head here. Push in up to the first knuckle and swirl the tip around, gently stretching. This takes time, try to get pleasurable sounds from your partner, watch their body language, and slowly go deeper. Talk to your partner. Tell them not to worry if they feel like they have to go to the bathroom. This is almost always because they now have something in their ass. It feels weird the first time something is going in and not out!

    Give this finger play a lot of time, gently open them, one finger deep, swirling around slowly, gently in and out, then add another but just play with the tips in. Start over with what you did with one finger. If you get your partner moving with your hand, pushing back and moaning, great! Tell them to take deep breaths and push back. They may be holding their breath and not really thinking about it. Our body tends to tense up at new sensations.

    You may be tempted to rub your partner's clit to help her relax and get turned on, but remember, the hand that is going in your partner's ass should not get in or close to the vagina. Use your other hand or if you are not that dexterous, stay away from the vagina and clit until after the anal prep so you can either break telling them to stay put or use the anti-bacterial wipes. Use them thoroughly. You can always use a condom on your fingers for easier clean up and to help make sure there is no ass to vagina contact.

    So now your partner is stretched and ready. You have slowly helped the sphincter (ring of muscle inside the anus, towards the end of the rectum) relax. It is this ring of muscle that will offer the most resistance when you use your cock or dildo. Position them comfortably. This does not have to be doggy style but that position works well. You can have your partner on their back with pillows under their hips and legs up. This allows for eye contact, access to breasts and nipples, kissing, and watching your partner's face. Lube up your cock or dildo, use lots of lube!!!!

Hold your partner's cheeks apart and don't do this in the dark the first time. You need to see. Aim well and push just the head in slooooowly. Use very gentle in and out motions going in just a bit. Push deeper and as you feel the resistance of the sphincter, push past it. This is what will cause the most pain or discomfort. Be gentle; remind them to breathe and to push down or back. Go slow with gentle pushing, talk to your partner. Be encouraging. Telling them they are a dirty whore who loves being fucked in the ass can wait unless your partner is really feeling into it. Your partner is going to be worried about making a mess and all the new sensations, but mostly about the mess factor.

Once you have slowly pushed in, hold it for a little bit, talk to your partner, when you pull out is the feeling slick and easy? If not, apply more lube to the shaft. Once you feel your partner relax then things are good. They may say it feels weird, feels like they have to go to the bathroom, or that it hurts. Remind them they can use a safeword. Do not ignore the 'please stop', but ask them to relax, to give it a minute to allow their body to get used to the feeling. Rub their clit (clean hand please) to aid in relaxation, pull out so only the tip is in, then if they give you an okay proceed gently and slowly. Do not jump into wham bam, hard fucking like in the porno flicks. A good slow fuck is going to feel good to your cock because the ass is so tight. Go slow and use lots of clitoral stimulation. Anal orgasms are possible but you can save that goal for another time. Use clitoral stimulation to both relax your partner and so she gets pleasure. Remember you want her to like this so she will agree to do it again.

If you are a bit messy when you pull out, just shut up about it. You have towels and wipes there, use them. She will probably ask if she is messy and it will feel like she is, your dick just came out of her ass. Just say no, it's just lube and cum and wipe your partner clean.

Remember!!!

- Use lots of lube.
- Prep with your partner with your fingers.
- Wait for your partner to show signs of relaxation or pleasure.
- Keep towels at hand and anti-bacterial wipes.
- No ass to vagina or mouth. This spreads bad bacteria. It just isn't safe.
- Talk to your partner.
- Go slow, I mean really slow.
- Shut up about any clean up that is needed. "No baby, it's just lube, no mess."

Now if you have passed go and collected a green light for anal and you both want the fantasy or forced anal, have your partner wear a plug to get their muscles relaxed. They can push it in and out, toy with it, wear it for an hour or so and use it to stretch themselves out. Have them lube themselves up before hand. This does not mean you don't need lube on your cock or dildo. It just means your partner took care of anal foreplay and has already made themselves slick and ready. You can role play this with little imagination. Tone of voice, harshness of pushing in (WITH LUBE!!) using derogatory dirty talk, holding them down, etc. THIS IS ROLEPLAY a consensual act of sex.

If you wish for your partner to be focused on a punishment spanking and add another aspect by using anal while spanking then please still use lube and use your finger (note the use of singular finger) or a small plug. It doesn't take much to get a big sensation inside the ass. I do not feel the anal penetration should be the focus. The spanking which is heightened by the scolding and the use of a finger or small plug is okay IF your partner does not have anal on their hard limit list.

It is my hope that those searching for forced anal, anal rape, and anal punishment will take the time to read this. People, you want them to LIKE it. You will get much more anal sex if your partner likes it too. The use of anal during a punishment is okay if it is not on the hard limit list. Forced anal sex is rape. If you care for your sub, partner, spouse, don't do that to them. Really, just don't.

Understanding the Appeal of Spanking

Disclaimer: I am not a medical professional or sex therapist. Any information provided is my own opinion based on 10+ years of living a kinky lifestyle. Any activities mentioned are consensual. I am speaking of a pleasurable spanking here in most cases, not one for punishment.

So what is the big deal with spanking, and why does it turn so many people on?

First I want to address the psychological aspects of getting spanked. Not all people who enjoy spanking are heavy masochists, that is, people who enjoy pain. My wife is not, my play partner is. Some of them crave the power exchange. When I spank someone, they are relinquishing the power of controlling what happens to them over to me. Some seek the comfort spanking provides. The masochist can find safety and comfort through giving up power and control. They make themselves vulnerable and that is why trust is important.

Over the lap or over the knee spanking can be a very intimate act. Spanking a bare bottom with my bare hand adds an element of touch that is missing when I use a hairbrush or paddle. It is skin to skin contact, and there is also an aspect of closeness because I am holding onto my wife as I spank her. I don't do over the lap spanking with anyone but my wife. It is a comfortable position for both of us, and she can let go of the stress of life and the need to be in control and worry about responsibility for herself. It becomes my job. She turns it over to me. She is vulnerable but safe. It is freeing and it is bonding. Over the lap spanking with my wife often has the end result of orgasm unless it is a true punishment spanking. All spanking ends with holding her close and giving comfort. Even a punishment spanking can be pleasurable or at least freeing in the end because the person being punished has paid the price for the wrong they committed. They have been punished, the misdeed is over, they are 'good' again, and the misdeed is forgotten in the sense that the slate is wiped clean. The pain is good, and it has dissipated the stress or negativity.

Spanking can take away one's control as well so they are not responsible for the sexual arousal they feel or their kinky fantasies. Many people were programed as kids that sex is bad or dirty. All of the bad or naughty things happening to the person being spanked, isn't their 'fault'. If it is dirty or humiliating or wrong, well it's being forced on them. Remember forced is consensual here be it through pre spanking negotiation or within a power exchange relationship. One can be punished for all the nasty, slutty things they feel or desire. Yes, they enjoyed all the filthy things done to them but hey, it wasn't their fault. They were made to like it. Force here is consensual, but being punished for your filthy desires takes away the blame of enjoying those same dirty things.

The physical aspects of spanking differ in degree from person to person. For the person being spanked, there is often a release of endorphins resulting from the administering of pain. This confuses the pain and pleasure sensors in the body and can result in a euphoric feeling. The pain that is inflicted gives the masochist a high. It becomes pleasurable. This turns the spanking into something enjoyable. The pain feels good. Often if one is spanked to tears there is an emotional release. The floodgates open and all the stress bottled up inside rushes out. I have found that some cry as they orgasm. Again, it's the final and complete release found without the guilt.

Professional Dommes don't do sex, but the person who has a session with them gets an emotional and physical fulfillment none the less. Guilt may be released, humiliation given for feeling all those dirty things, many may go home and find sexual release after a session because it was sexually arousing, but the session gives them freedom to fulfill the sexual need. I knew a woman who saw her dominant once a month and he punished her hard for all the stuff she had screwed up on over the past month. Bad decisions, unsafe activities, careless actions, they were all erased by being punished. No sex was involved but she sure as hell went home and masturbated.

Why do I spank? What does it do for me? Not all spankings are sexual for me. With my play partner, I spank for the emotional release and the sadistic high. I am sadistic and dominant. I enjoy the power rush I get when someone has given me control of their body. I get a rush from making them feel. I control what they feel. I can make the feeling more intense depending on our needs by using words, restraints, implements, and different amounts of force. I take my partner through the gambit of a wide range of emotions, and with my wife, sexual arousal. I control everything she feels. Is it pleasure, pain, or a mix of both? It's all up to me. Spanking my wife is very sexually arousing for me, and unless it is a punishment spanking, it's more like foreplay. That's why even though my need for sadism doesn't get completely fulfilled because she isn't a huge pain lover, it does give me pleasure because the power given to me and the act in which I take power from her as she lays helpless over my lap, still is erotic and stimulating.

With my play partner, I know he is a huge masochist, and so I get pleasure from giving him what he needs. I do not use my hand to spank my play partner, but that is just me, others may differ. I do not get sexually aroused, but I do get an adrenaline rush and it provides stress release. I akin the S/m play with my play partner to recreation. It is an enjoyable activity for us both and we take different things from it. Again though, it is not sexual, but it is most definitely fun. It took me a good long while to come to terms with my inner sadist, but that is a topic for another day. Just remember that consent is the key.

If you are looking to add spanking make sure there is communication beforehand. I don't recommend trying to piss off your lover so they spank you. Many people would feel huge guilt for hurting their partner after the fact if it wasn't talked about before. Remember that your partner may be reluctant and may not get a great feeling the first time because they are too worried about really hurting you. Talking is a must, trust is a must, consent is a must, and aftercare or emotional and physical support for the one spanked is a must. I cuddle my wife, I provide my play partner with water, chocolate or other little bit of sugar or protein, I watch over him until I am sure he is steady and clear headed, I make sure both are warm, and can sit or relax. I accept my responsibility for their care before, during, and after they experience the emotional and physical feelings that result from spanking.

If you are interested in reading about spanking and play session examples between two consenting adults that will go from the beginning of a scene through the end and include all aspects that are important including the aftercare, you can find them in two of my books. They are the BDSM collections. They are NOT like 50 Shades. They are real, and many may be deemed harsh by those who are new. That said, these are scenes I have done, the way I play, and both participants are getting their needs met. They are consensual and wanted by both people.

You may disagree or have different reactions to spanking or giving spankings. This book is intended to give my views from my personal stand point. I am not speaking for everyone. Comments or questions can be sent to my blog or the email listed in the front of this book. Your views are welcomed and encouraged.

Styles and Reasons for Spanking

Disclaimer – This chapter is intended for consenting adults only. I hold no responsibility for anyone's actions after reading this book. Proceed at your own risk. I am not liable. I do not recommend spanking without knowing a good deal about it, and knowing how an implement feels before you use it on someone. Communication beforehand is vital. Any actions done after reading this book are the sole responsibility of the reader. Be safe, sane, and consensual. Spanking someone without their consent is abuse.

I will begin with the punishment spanking because like all punishment, I feel it's better to get it over with. I am speaking of a real punishment spanking, not one done for the enjoyment of both parties. Punishment spankings are very different than those I give my wife during foreplay, a BDSM session, or for bonding. Punishment holds no joy for me, and is very much disliked by my wife. That is the huge difference between punishment and 'funishment'. Please remember, do not punish your partner when you are angry! Send them to the corner until you cool off or set a later time. Make sure they are aware the spanking is coming.

When one is going to spank their partner for punishment, corner time before or after (I prefer before) can heighten the punishment. Standing in the corner, bottom bare, thinking about what is to come and thinking about why the punishment is coming, can be almost as bad as the pain of the spanking, but in a different way. One is mental, you are addressing the brain and emotions. You are making the one who has earned a punishment think about what they did and really have time to regret their poor behavior. When I send my wife to the corner, I tell her why, what is going to occur afterward, but often do not tell her for how long. This puts her in the proper frame of mind and I know she is focused on the punishment and only the punishment. I have her bottom (or all of her depending on if it's winter), bare, her nose pressed to the wall, hands at her sides. Absolutely no speaking and no moving until I tell her it's time for her spanking. Some prefer to make their partner press a penny to the wall with their nose to ensure proper positioning.

    I give punishment spankings in three different positions, the first can be bent over the edge of the bed or a chair, arms outstretched, holding on, legs apart, the second, on the spanking bench, wrist cuffs and ankle cuffs on to inhibit movement. The third and the one I prefer and use most is her over my lap. We do this with my sitting on the bed leaning against the headboard. I prefer to have her lie across my lap when on the bed because it gives her a steady place to lie, and I don't have to worry about her slipping. Some prefer to have their partner over their lap or knee in a chair to keep them unbalanced; I would rather be stable and be able to hold her around the waist to keep her in place.

    The position of bent over the chair or bed is used when the implement is a belt or cane. I need a wider swing range than I can have over my lap. If your partner is a big masochist the belt may not be a good implement. My wife is not. A hard lashing with the belt on her bottom and upper thighs is truly a punishment for her. Many people find the belt erotic and my wife actually can, but not if it is swung with the intent of really hurting. If one wishes to use a cane, they need their partner in this kind of position or on a spanking bench. You cannot use a cane in the over the knee or lap position, or at least I can't.

When I punish my wife over my lap in our bed I use the wooden hairbrush. This implement is used only for punishment and stings like hell. I stroke her back and bare bottom before proceeding, telling her once again why she is receiving the spanking, then I wrap my arm around her waist. I spank hard, though it doesn't take much to make my point clear. As I spank I speak to her. I always tell her that I love her but that the behavior is not acceptable. A finger inserted into your partner's bottom as you scold can really drive the point home. I spank one cheek five or so times then move to the other cheek and back again. I may spank over and over in one spot as I scold. I spank the center and lower bottom, not the top, and I aim for a few in the crease where her thighs meet her bottom. I will use my hand to stretch this skin and open the crease up a bit to emphasize my point. The number of spanks and the force of the blows depend on what I am spanking her for. Some spank to tears, I do not. My wife hardly ever cries. Spanking to tears is more spanks than I think she could take. She could use her safeword and I would accept it, BUT she never would during a punishment.

Afterwards, I stroke her back, bottom, and hair and speak softly. Once it is over, the transgression is done, she is forgiven. When she is calm, I pull her up so we can cuddle and tell her I love her and that she is a good girl. Aftercare is very important. I do not send her to the corner after a punishment spanking. Again, your mileage may vary.

A 'funishment' spanking can be done in any number of ways and with any number of implements. It is meant to be enjoyable to both parties. Some people like to build up with some type of fantasy such as naughty school girl, a Victorian scene, boss and secretary, you get the idea. Whatever gets you going, the key here is that you PRETEND the spanking is a punishment, but it truly isn't. You can add scolding and name calling, perhaps spanking your partner for being a dirty little slut or so on. When I used such derogatory terms with my wife, they are said with love. She knows I do not think she really is a slut, whore, etc. This is part of the build-up. I am not into humiliation, and my dirty talk isn't done with that intent.

Whatever your choice, build up the scene. Give a warm up spanking mixed with rubs on the back, bottom, or if you are intimate with your partner, between the legs or on the genitals. If your partner is aroused or wet you can scold them for being dirty and nasty and "How dare they become aroused when they have been so bad?" I usually hand spank first, and then the focus is on using implements we both enjoy. I am very mindful of her pain/pleasure peak. I do push her a bit, but not too much because as I said, she is not a pain puppy.

Her 'funishment' spankings are done in a more sensual way with a slow build up to the burn and I don't stay long at the height of her tolerance. I use what is called a horse bat most when she is over my lap. You can find good quality implements at The Horse Tack Co. online. Fetish stores and adult toy sites really over price their items. For crops, leather slappers, and whips, you should try the horse tack places. Farm and Fleet has a good selection as well. Just don't go out and start trying them on your partner in the store!

    A good quality spanking is a mix of build-up and other touches. Maybe a scratching of the nails, rubbing, little fast pats then up to harder and sharper, stingy and painful to get the endorphins rushing, then back to rubbing, squeezing again. My play partner is male and there is no erotic touch, but I do rub his back and scratch at the welts I leave with my canes and such, but the build-up, then slow down, then build up is still important no matter what pain level you build-up to. Touch is important, don't just whale away on and on with no change. Cover the entire bottom, all the fleshy soft parts, and inner thighs if you wish for a more intimate spanking, back of thighs if you are going for more pain.

    Words are sexy and enhance the experience. You can scold, talk dirty, demand answers if you are playing the role of the angry partner who is meting out punishment. Mix things up with sexual arousal if you are both okay with that. Spanking can be foreplay for sex, an activity in its own, a well scripted scene, or a serious punishment. Just remember, even punishment spanking are consensual. All play should be preceded by conversation unless you and your partner have been playing for a good long while, and safewords should always be respected, and aftercare is a must, ESPECIALLY after a discipline spanking.

So...
- Decide on the type of spanking you wish or need to give.
- Decide on the implement or implements you are going to use and have them within reach.
- Decide on how you will position your partner.
- Decide on the hows of your partner. How will they be clothed? (Spanking on the panties and then pulling them down is hot). How will your partner be supported especially if their knees get weak?

How will you make sure you can cuddle after? How much of a masochist is your partner? How intimate are the two of you? Will the spanking be the build-up to sex? If so, how will you reposition to the place you will be having sex? How much time do you have? Is it enough for one implement or several? Is there time for aftercare?

Decide on the tone of the spanking. If it is for punishment, make sure your partner knows what they did wrong.

If you punish to tears, make sure you dry those tears and let your partner know they have been forgiven and redeemed.

During aftercare, are you going to rub lotion on your partner's blazing bottom? There are creams meant for numbing the penis so a guy can stay hard longer that work well to soothe a punished bottom. Have water or

some other drink without booze at hand. Make sure you have a way to keep your partner warm.
    Make sure you have consent!

The Ins and Outs of BDSM Gatherings

As promised, I will speak on the ins and outs of a CFNM (Clothed Female, Nude Male), but I have decided to include what the different types of kink gatherings are.

Munch – A munch is a term meaning an informal get together of people interested in kink. Here in Milwaukee we have various different munches that appeal to a wide variety of people. Munches are held at a public place, and there is no BDSM play. Dress is to be street legal and the conversation topics are as diverse as the people who attend them.

We have munches or a subs dinner for just submissive types, a monthly dinner for all that includes a meal, a weekly munch held at a bar that could technically be called a slosh because there is no food. Typically we just use the term munch. And we have a monthly munch for everyone at a bar in a bowling alley. There are vanillas there as well. We generally look like any other group of people.

A munch is NOT;

A place for any play.

An event where dominants should expect other submissives to wait on them or be submissive to them. If someone is not your submissive then don't expect them to act as if they were.

Munches are not organized to be any type of pick up or dating help. Just because you are at a munch doesn't mean you act as if the pretty lady next to you wants to be hit on or played with. Act with the manners that are required for all social functions. Go to meet people, not hunt for a partner.

Events – There are many large events around the country. These are normally held at big hotels. The days are spent in classes on every type of kink you can think of, there are other fun things like pageants and shows, and the evenings host large dungeon space with lots of equipment to play on. There are vendors to buy goodies from as well.

People tend to dress in their kinky best at night for the dungeon, but toned down for the day. In general you must be street legal until you pass through the event security and into the event space. Once inside most anything goes. We love big events. They are a chance to immerse yourself into all things kink for an entire weekend, connect with old friends and make new ones, as well as learn something.

Events can also be camping. We have several of those around the Midwest that involve lots of hedonistic fun in the woods. Naked outdoor frolics. We have a special camping event we absolutely love each summer. No tents for us, cabins and a lodge to play in as well as private woods and lake.

Informational Gatherings – These are meetings that can take place in people's homes, the local play space, public venues, or places such as a kink friendly store. They are meant to teach or discuss a particular subject. It may be on a type of play or relationship. They can be to teach rope skills, learn about wax play, relationship issues that are unique to BDSM, and everything else. Fetlife has tons of groups to find these and munches in your area.

Private Play Parties – These are just that with the emphasis on private. Don't expect an invite until people know you. We have a dungeon in our basement but NO ONE gets invited or through our door unless we know them well and know they are safe and sane. Some people come for socializing, some to play, some to watch and learn.

Some parties are specialized like the CFNM's we have had. Again, no one gets invited that we don't know very well. This is for the men serving and for our lady guests. The day will consist of the ladies arriving to be seated and tended by their male nude server with beverages, appetizers, and a chance for us ladies to chit chat a bit. In general the guys are seen but not heard. It is a formal event. The men have been taught what is expected. No glass should go under 1/2 full, no dirty plate left in our vicinity, each course is announced, service is top notch. I require bowties and allow shoes.

Once everyone arrives, we have our formal dinner. The men serve their lady each course, again keeping an eye on anything needed. I have one of our close guy friends acting as major domo to keep the kitchen well run so my wife can relax.

After dinner we have games. Target practice where the men's cocks are pulled through the center of a bull's-eye and we practice shooting rubber bands trying to get a direct hit. The men blow party horns when one of the ladies hits her target. A score is kept, prizes given.

Ring toss – We toss rings around the men's cocks. The men are required to keep themselves hard. If their lady wants to touch and help, that is allowed. Again, a score is kept.

Deck the Dick – We had great fun with this. I provided all sorts of craft materials including wiggly eyes and feathers and the ladies decorated their servant's dick. The pictures are hilarious and can be seen on my profile of Inaralee on Fetlife.com.

Afterward foot massages are given. This is the best part for me! Also, the men can earn chips for good service and they can turn them in for a turn on the spanking bench or cross.

All men fill out a consent form that speaks of their limits and all play must be negotiated. The ladies are told ahead of time about their server. In my mind you have to have a low ratio of women to men for success. As the hostess it is also my job to make sure there is no violation of consent with any play.

That's about it. My parties don't focus on humiliation. We all have fun. A lot goes into the planning. I put sticky notes all over the kitchen to keep the guys on track with their duties. It's not that they would dare slack off, it's because I don't want to be bothered with questions during the party. I train them, we plan out the menu, Beauty and I decide on the fun and games, and last but not least, I turn up the heat. No one will have fun if my guys freeze, and dangly bits tend to shrivel if it's cold.

Power Exchange Means Give and Take

My wife is my collared submissive and TiH. I plan her schedule, assign her tasks, give her structure, teach her how I want things to be done, nurture, sometimes fuss and nag, and I make all the decisions in our lives and our relationships. She knows that I will take charge in any situations that will affect us. I will take care of anything bad. I will support her when she wants to try something, I will say yes or no when she wants something. I will tell her what it is she should do. All of these things can lead to a misconception about a power exchange relationship and how it makes the TiH, submissive, or slave less capable. I fall under that same misconception sometimes too, but when I do, I'm wrong. I shouldn't be scared for her or think she will struggle out in the world without me; Beauty is so much stronger than that. Our relationship has helped us both be well armed for the stupidity and general mess of the world.

Being submissive and not making your own decisions in a relationship and in life does not make the submissive less able to take care of themselves. Just because you want someone else to lead and to feel taken care of, doesn't mean you can't do it. It means you would rather not do it. That's a big difference. Being submissive does not mean being weak. It's the opposite really, it means she is strong enough and sure enough in herself to pick the right person to hand her life over to and trust her submission with.

A power exchange relationship should be one that includes well rounded domination. You are exchanging power, not taking it away, and not making it all about the dominant. When a dominant takes the power, they are supposed to give something back. Each person in the exchange gets what they need. It is not one sided.

When I take away the decision making, I give my wife the freedom to focus on being the best she can be in our relationship.

When I take over the daily running of our lives with schedules and expectations, I give her the freedom to let go of the stress of running a household, paying the bills, how to keep from being overwhelmed because it is broken into bite size pieces that can be handled.

When I am strict and punish her for not doing as required or for bad behavior, I am giving the structure she very much needs in order for her world to be a place where she is loved, guided, and made to feel secure.

When I give orders, she gives a place to call home that is a place where I can relax and leave my burdens at the door.

When I give decision making, she gives me a life void of the little thing that take time and make life harder. I don't have to worry about putting gas in the car, going to the bank, buying groceries, feeding and cleaning up after the pets, driving when I'm exhausted, running out of toilet paper, or a million other little things.

When I give structure, she gives a well-run day that my type A personality needs and the specific schedule she needs. Daily rituals, dinner on time, bedtime rituals.

When I give safety and security, she gives nurturing and love.

When I give strength and empowerment, she gives it right back. We help each other cope when one of us can't be strong.

When I give ownership, she gets a place in my life that is all hers. She can take pride in knowing I love her enough to want her for life, and that I will always be here for her.

We exchange the power. We give and take love. We give and take nurturing, we give and take security. We give and take lives that allow us peace. We give and take what each other needs to find comfort. We give and take support.

I do not dominate to overpower. I do not dominate so I can always have things my way. I do not dominate so I can force my wife to do things she doesn't want to do. I do not dominate to crush, break, or smother. I lift her up, I empower her, I do my best to give her self-confidence.

Submissive does not mean weak. Submissive does not mean unable. Submissive does not mean helpless. Submissive does not mean messed up or broken.

I am the one who had to have all the pets' schedules typed up when Beauty was going to be gone a few days. I am the one who needed dinners made and put in the freezer. I am the one who had to be shown where basic stuff was kept in the house. I am the one who felt panicky when it was time for her to go and kept saying be safe, be smart, and be careful. She could and did do it because she is a capable adult. My dominance has helped her grow. I have helped her be equipped for the world by being in a relationship where we give and take the best of ourselves.

So I guess it goes back to the thing I keep preaching about to those who want to be dominant. It isn't all about you, and in some ways having a TiH makes you less powerful. My wife takes care of me, and I take care of us. I may be the dominant, but her role is vitally important. Owning or having a TiH, a submissive, or a slave is a responsibility but it's also something to be treasured.

I am not the great and powerful Oz, I am the person behind the curtain who works all the whistles and bells. I can make good things happen, and even to do great things, but I am not doing it alone. Beauty is my dials, levers, and gadgets. My life is made more wonderful because Beauty is in it, and her life is more wonderful because I am in hers. So now I ask you, who do you think is the dependent one in the relationship? I'd say we both are, and I'm not ashamed in the least by my answer.

Domestic discipline and power exchange relationships done properly, makes for two very happy people. I wouldn't live my life any other way, and it is my sincere hope that others find their way down the same path that Beauty and I walk.

Jolynn Raymond
Taken In Hand
December 2013

Notes:

Printed in Great Britain
by Amazon